CONCILIUM OPHTHALMOLOGICUM UNIVERSALE

PERIMETRIC STANDARDS

and

PERIMETRIC GLOSSARY

of the International Council of Ophthalmology

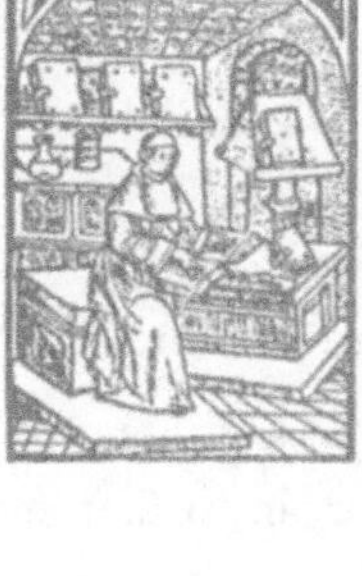

Dr. W. Junk bv Publishers The Hague/Boston/London 1979

Softcover reprint of the hardcover 1st edition 1979

ISBN 978-94-009-9641-0 ISBN 978-94-009-9639-7 (eBook)
DOI 10.1007/ 978-94-009-9639-7

PERIMETRIC STANDARDS, 1978

Committee: Jay M. ENOCH (U.S.A., chairman of the IPS[1] R.G. on Standards, *editor*), and (alphabetically) Elfriede AULHORN (GFR), André DUBOIS-POULSEN (France), Frank FANKHAUSER (Switzerland), Allan FRIEDMANN (UK), Erik GREVE (The Netherlands, secretary of the IPS[1]), H. HARMS (GFR) and Guy VERRIEST (Belgium).

Members of this Ad Hoc Drafting Committee to prepare an International Perimetric Standard were selected at a meeting of the R.G.[1] on Standards of the IPS[1], September 19, 1976, Tübingen, West Germany. This meeting was held at the Universitäts-Augenklinik, Bonn-Venusberg, West Germany, on November 11-12, 1977. The Ad Hoc Committee wishes to express its appreciation to Prof. Best of Bonn for his cooperation and many acts of kindness during the preparation of this draft proposal.

The Research Group on Standards would like to thank the many individuals who have offered thoughtful and constructive criticisms. Many of their proposed changes have been incorporated in this document.

[1] R.G., Research Group; IPS, International Perimetric Society

CONTENTS

IPS PERIMETRIC STANDARDS, 1978

1. Definitions of Perimetry and of the Visual Field

Perimetry is the measurement of visual functions of the eye at topographically defined loci in the visual field. The visual field is that portion of the external environment of the observer wherein the steadily fixating eye(s) can detect visual stimuli.

2. Need for Specifications and Tolerances

The fundamental purpose of standardization is to provide a common framework for measurement. This allows exchange and comparison of information obtained at different times and in different places. If a common measurement scheme can be achieved, then development upon that base can proceed in an orderly manner.

In perimetry few standards exist and certain of these are imperfectly specified. This situation needs to be rectified.

Specification also implies consideration of tolerances. Tolerances include instrument setting accuracy as well as measurement accuracy. Because tolerances in a clinical office are not comparable with those achievable in a research laboratory, an effort will be made to set standards which define conditions where small errors do not significantly alter results or interpretations of data.

3. Applicability of this Standard

This standard is written for all individuals engaged in perimetry and especially for clinicians for use in their offices, departments, and clinics. It is directed also towards the manufacturer who provides visual field test equipment. These standards also set minimum criteria for reporting research results. The goal is to set a reasonable minimum set of standards for testing of the visual field. Note that different requirements or strategies may be needed for different tasks.

4. Specifications of Magnitudes and Units

This committee makes use of the International System of Units published by the International Bureau of Weights and Measures (Le Système International d'Unités, 1970, OFFILIB, 48 Rue Gay-Lussac, F-75005, Paris, France, Revised edition 1977). See also: The International System of Units, NBS Special Publication 330, 1977, U.S. Department of Commerce, National Bureau of Standards, U.S. Government Printing Office, Washington, D.C. 20402 (SD Catalogue No. C13.10:330/4). Supplemental use is made of the Vocabulary of the Commission Internationale de l'Eclairage (International Lighting Vocabulary of the Commission Internationale de l'Eclairage, 3rd ed., 1970, Bureau Central de la CIE, 4 Avenue du Recteur Poincaré, F-75016, Paris, France).

In the Proceedings (Acta) of the XXIInd International Ophthalmological Congress, Paris, 1974, p. 78 and 93, the Concilium Ophthalmologicum Universale published recommendations regarding the use of the International System of Units in ophthalmological practice.

There is on record an earlier international standard on perimetry which was published by the XIII Concilium Ophthalmologicum 1929, Hollandia, N.V. Boek- en Steendrukkerij, Edward IJdo, Leiden, 9 pages. The present document is meant to supercede this earlier standard.

Recently the Committee on Vision, the National Research Council, National Academy of Sciences of the United States of America published the "First Interprofessional Standard for Visual Field Testing," National Academy of Sciences, Washington, D.C., 1975. Certain aspects of the present document are based upon this publication.

5. Photometric Specification

For proper control of visual stimuli in perimetry, provision of one or more light sources is necessary. That is, the background, test stimuli, and all supplementary targets or display fields need to be specified photometrically.

The specification of visual stimuli is complex. Properly, radiant energy determinations should be made, followed by suitable luminous conversions for different field areas and stimulus conditions. For most practical clinical situations the IPS recommends that the visual stimulus in perimetry be specified in luminance units measured at the center of the entrance pupil of the eye. The visual stimulus is essentially defined by this luminance, the direction of the stimulus in the field of view and the area of the entrance pupil of the eye. Since we often cannot control pupil size in the clinical environment, the least we can achieve is to specify luminance at the center of the entrance pupil of the eye, and to request the examiner to record this luminance and the entrance pupil size at the time of the measurement.

In certain conditions special additional calibration requirements exist, *e.g.*, for short duration or colored stimuli.

We ask the manufacturer to specify the operating conditions of his instrument. Ideally this would include the complete specifications of lamps, filters (including transmission curves), and desired operating conditions. Luminance at the center of the entrance pupil of the eye should be specified for defined operating conditions of properly centered light sources and associated optics. Similarly, the spectral distribution at the entrance pupil of the eye should be defined. In addition, definition of desired operating color temperature and CIE coordinates is highly desirable. A simple scheme for assuring that the instrument is functioning within reasonable tolerances of these specified values should be provided. Included would be some test of luminance and/or indication for replacement of light sources.

The international unit of luminance is the candela per meter squared, cd/m^2 or $cd.m^{-2}$. Other units are now regarded as obsolete. Although strictly speaking not the same units[2], conversion to apostilb and millilambert values can be made using the following relationships:

$$10/\pi \text{ candela/m}^2 = 1 \text{ millilambert} = 10 \text{ apostilbs},$$
$$\text{where } 10/\pi = 3.183 \text{ (approximate)}.$$

While this group would prefer luminance measurement of perimetric devices by objective small field test instruments, an acceptable alternative would be to provide a measure convertible into luminance at the center of the entrance pupil of the eye.

6. Background or Adapting Luminance

A. Specification of luminance

For routine perimetric instruments used in clinical offices it is recommended that a value of background luminance be chosen such that it is photopic and it falls within that range of background luminances over which the Weber fraction remains constant, *i.e.*, $\Delta L/L_B$ = constant.[3] ΔL is defined as

[2] See discussion in the recently published U.S. Standard relative to this point.

[3] For example, see E. Aulhorn, H. Harms, and M. Raabe, Documenta Ophthal. *20*, 538-556, 1966; and J. Enoch, Physiology (Chapter 3, pp 202-289) in A. Sorsby, Modern Ophthalmology, Vol I, First Ed., 1963; and the recent U.S.A. Standard referenced above.

the just detectable luminance difference between test target and background,[4] and L_B is background luminance (also see section on contrast). The proposed background level is generally higher than that found in perimeters in use today. This setting criterion is recommended because (a) it requires less sensitive calibration equipment, (b) it is less sensitive to modest fluctuations (or changes) in light source output, (c) the result is less dependent upon modest variations in eye pupil size, (d) visual functions are tested at clearly defined photopic levels, and (e) fixation control is easier than at low luminance adaptation levels.

If this background luminance cannot be achieved, it is recommended that for routine office purposes no less than 10 candelas/m^2 be used. A background luminance of 10 candelas/m^2 is below, but near the level where $\Delta L/L_B$ = constant over an extended range of values.

Other light or adaptation levels offer advantages. Lower levels may provide an extended range of contrast values for testing, cataract patients may be better evaluated, and rod anomalies may be more effectively studied, *etc.* Thus, where adequate calibration capability exists and careful studies are conducted to rule out loss of confidence due to increased measurement variance, lower photopic or mesopic background luminance levels can serve a useful purpose. Similarly, higher background luminance values can be useful in tests of the visual fatigue factor or for the development of color perimetric tests.

Thus the IPS recommends that instruments be constructed to be capable of calibration over a range of values. The IPS suggests that the standard be a minimum test condition rather than a limiting condition. We encourage careful research on this rather complex and crucial set of questions. We recognize that stability of determinations in special disease conditions, *e.g.*, glaucoma, cataract, chorioretinal degenerations, optic neuropathies, *etc.*, may require use of special or specific background luminance levels and spacial purpose instruments suitable for advanced diagnostic laboratories.

B. Preadaptation conditions

It is highly desirable that the patient be adapted to the luminance of the background field before commencement of the perimetric test. A longer

[4] The specification of ΔL is somewhat arbitrary, because the probability of detecting the test target varies between 0 and 1 over a small range of luminances. ΔL is commonly specified as the luminance increment or difference corresponding to a detection probability of 0.5 (50% frequency-of-seeing).

time period of preadaptation to this field is necessary for lower background luminance levels. It should also be longer if the patient enters the examination chamber from an intensely luminous environment. It is desirable that the manufacturer and examiner determine the light adaptation period which provides relatively stable response for the instrument and conditions used. Preadaptation conditions can also be important when testing individuals manifesting certain types of pathology.

C. Diffusely reflecting surface
It is desirable that the background field be a diffusely reflecting surface, *i.e.*, a non-glossy surface which at least approximates Lambert's Law.

7. Specification of the location of an Object in the Visual Field

A polar coordinate system should be used when defining (a) the half-meridian and (b) the eccentricity of the center of the test target, both expressed in degrees. The zero degree half-meridian is defined to the right of the patient (as seen by the patient). The specified half-meridian then proceeds counterclockwise through 360° about the fixation target (as seen by the patient). The fixation point is defined at having zero degree eccentricity. This assumes the patient has normal fixation.

This system does not allow fine specification of the *area* of a scotoma or of an isopter because of non-linearity of representation,[5] except in the case of a hemisphere where proportional solid angles are present. This requires the center of the entrance pupil of the eye to lie at the center of curvature of the hemisphere. In this special case, two equal solid angles located at different loci in the visual field subtend equal areas on the surface of the hemisphere. This condition does not exist if a flat test surface is used for examination of the visual field, *e.g.*, when a tangent screen is employed. The same statement may be applied to the cartographic deformation of the field as expressed on a flat sheet of paper. There exist cartographic projections which attempt to represent areas proportionately.

It is highly desirable to keep the tolerances for location, registration, and replication of test object position within narrow limits. If this cannot be achieved, the reliability of subsequent determinations is limited, especially for static (target not moving) perimetry. Accuracy is limited by the size and nature of the fixation target, the stability of patient fixation,

[5] Distinguish between ability to specify a location and an area.

and the mechanical capabilities of the perimetric device.[6] In turn, these factors influence the selection of the smallest useful target size.

Optimal fixation targets have not yet been defined. This is an important question which needs clarification through research. Obviously, it is desirable to monitor patient fixation directly. When central vision is impaired, special fixation targets or displays are often needed.

It is desirable that measured test points should be indicated on the test record in an obvious manner. Clearly the more points tested, the better the characterization of the visual field. The more repetitions of evaluations made at a single point, the greater the reliability of the determination. It is desirable that one or more points be evaluated more than once in order to define the approximate reliability of the test. It is desirable that interpolation or analysis techniques employed be clearly defined.

8. Target Specification (non-photometric)

A. Size, distance, and form

Ideally target dimensions should be specified in terms of the solid angle subtended at the center of the entrance pupil of the eye and measured in steradians. Practically, this is not done, nor do we recommend such designation as essential at this time.

A conceptually simpler scheme is the specification of the diameter of the target in terms of visual angle subtended at the center of the entrance pupil of the eye. This assumes that a round target is located at the point of fixation. If the target is not round, the diameter of the equivalent round target subtending the same area at the point of fixation may be used. Target diameters should be expressed in degrees, minutes, and seconds of arc. It is highly desirable to specify test target distance from the eye, because luminance is dependent on test distance for perimetric test targets of small dimension. (The same is not true for extended background fields.) Thus, for proper specification, it is highly desirable that both angular subtense and target distance be specified. Other factors, such as image blur resulting from several causes, also make specification of target distance desirable (see below, Image sharpness). As an example of proper specification, a

[6] Lens factors also influence accuracy of location and re-location of a target in the visual field. Apparent location of a target is influenced by power and centration of the lens correction, vertex distance, base curve and lens thickness. It is desirable that the lens(es) used and the vertex distance be noted. There is an advantage in keeping vertex distance small.

target may subtend 6' of arc (angular diameter) at a 330 millimeter test distance.

Alternatively, specification of the tangent of the angle subtended at the ceter of the entrance pupil of the eye for a target located at the fixation point has been widely used.

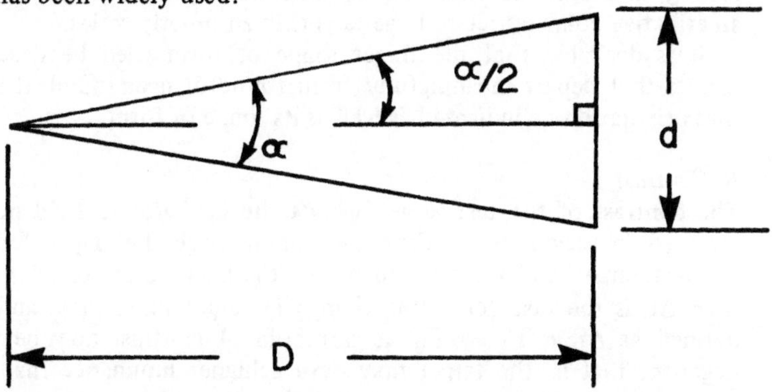

Fig. 1. $\frac{d}{D} = 2 \tan (\alpha/2)$

This measure is expressed as a fraction, the diameter (d) of the target in millimeters divided by the distance of the fixation point from the eye (D) in millimeters (*e.g.*, 2 mm white/1000 mm). Of the two schemes (the angle subtended plus the test distance versus the tangent fraction) the angle subtended and test distance is the preferred form of representation because it is conceptually simpler to compare angular subtense of targets on two different test instruments. Thus, the IPS recommends the specification of equivalent[7] test target diameter and distance as follows:

(a) minutes of arc diameter at (b) millimeters test distance. In publications this form is preferred. Other systems may be used if a logical scheme is formulated and if conversion to the above preferred form is provided.

When a tangent screen is used, and targets are displayed from the point of fixation, the angular subtenses, the solid angle subtended by the target, and the effective test distance are all altered. If a projector is used with a tangent screen, its center of projection must effectively be placed as near as possible to the location of the test eye in order to minimize distorting

[7]The use of equivalence is only valid for targets which approximate round shapes.

effects and blur. When tangent screens are used (or other perimetric devices) every effort should be made to make background luminance as uniform as possible.

It is desirable that a number of different size targets be available for testing, and that the visual angles subtended by these targets extend from an effective point source to large targets in an orderly series.

It is desirable that the target shape or form used be described. For targets that depart meaningfully from round or near round, it is desirable that orientation be indicated as well as its shape or form.

B. Contrast

The contrast of the test target against the background field may be represented in various ways, depending upon usage. Let L_T = luminance of the test target, and L_B = luminance of the background or adapting field,[8] then ΔL is the just detectable change in target luminance, and would be defined as $\Delta L = L_T - L_B$ at threshold. A contrast may be positive or negative, that is, the target may have a higher luminance than the background (positive contrast) or the darker than the background (negative contrast). All of the following formats have been used to describe contrast = C:

(a₁) $$C = \frac{L_T - L_B}{L_B}$$ (Recommended)

(a₂) $$C = \frac{|L_T - L_B|}{L_B}$$ [9]

(a₃) $$C_T = \frac{\Delta L}{L_B},$$ C_T = contrast at threshold (Recommended)

(b) $$C = \frac{L_T}{L_B}$$

(c) $$C = \frac{L_T - L_B}{L_T + L_B} = \frac{L_T - L_B}{2\left(\frac{L_T + L_B}{2}\right)}, \text{ where } \left(\frac{L_T + L_B}{2}\right) = \text{mean luminance}$$

NOTE: In a projection perimeter, ΔL is the projected incremental field and the luminance at the pointed tested $L_T = \Delta L + L_B$. Negative contrast, *i.e.*, a darker target against a brighter background, is rarely used in perimetry, but is commonly used in conjunction with visual acuity charts.

[8] That which follows assumes that L_B is greater than zero.

[9] $|X|$ symbol denotes absolute value, i.e., a value without sign.

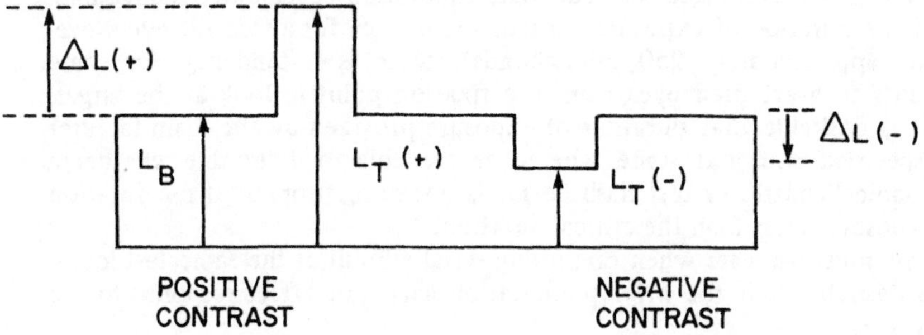

Fig. 2.

In routine perimetry form a_1 or a_3 is the recommended usage. For simplicity of design most tests performed use positive contrast. Form c is often used as a description of modulation in contrast sensitivity functions. Form a_3 is also known as the Weber fraction. As the increment or contrast threshold, form a_1 is equivalent to a_3. Since many forms exist for expression of contrast, it is desirable that the form employed be indicated.

C. Duration of presentation

1. *Non-moving or static target(s) (here we only consider a single presentation of the test target).* The response of the visual system changes with duration of exposure of a visual stimulus. The exposure time at which this transition occurs is known as the critical duration. The critical duration is about 100 milliseconds, and varies with several factors, including test target locus in the field, target size, background field luminance and pathology.

For exposures shorter than the critical duration,

$$\Delta L \times \text{Duration of exposure} = \text{Constant};$$

while for durations of exposure longer than the critical duration,

$$\Delta L = \text{Constant}.$$

Obviously the latter is a less demanding test situation for calibration as one less parameter needs to be specified in the test instrument. Shorter durations may be advantaged, but adequate calibration capacibility is advisable.

If the duration of exposure exceeds the latency for a saccadic eye movement (approximately 250 milliseconds), there is a tendency for some patients to avert their eyes from the fixation point to look at the target.

It is desirable that duration of exposure provided by the manufacturer be specified and that some scheme be available to determine whether a mechanical shutter or test flash device is operating properly if the duration of exposure is less than the critical duration.

One must use care when presenting serial stimuli at the same test locus. It is desirable that the prior presentation shall not affect response to the later ones.

2. *Moving or kinetic targets.* If the target or stimulus is moved, as in kinetic perimetry, the most important point is the stability of rate of movement, *i.e.,* a fixed angular velocity, initially and at the time of re-examination, Some perimetrists use a different strategy, *e.g.,* a somewhat slower rate of movement, in the central field. In most instances the target is moved from non-seeing to seeing. Other strategies may be used to fit specific needs. In recording and/or reporting results it is desirable (to the extent possible) that test conditions employed be described. Detectability of a moving target is dependent upon test target luminance and/or contrast, area, direction, and rate of movement. The measured results are subject to meaningful variation if such factors are not properly controlled. The specification of optimal test conditions is a complex question requiring further research. Thus, at this time, the IPS does not recommend any single desired rate of movement or test strategy. In so stating, the IPS in no way means to underestimate the importance of kinetic perimetry.

D. Image sharpness

One of the least appreciated variables in visual field testing is the blur of the retinal image of the test target. Many factors affect image blur. Appropriate optical correction to the test distance is needed especially for small test targets. This correction will vary with presbyopia, the use of miotics, cycloplegics, and in the presence of many forms of pathology, *etc.*

9. Color Perimetry

When reporting data, it is highly desirable to specify the observer's task, whether it be just detection or a judgment of hue and saturation of the target.

In color perimetry we recommend that both target and background field radiance and luminance be specified at the center of the entrance pupil of the eye. In anticipation of the development of new color perimetric tests, the IPS recommends a general increase in background and target luminance levels; spectral specification in the plane of the entrance pupil of light sources and stimuli (including the properties of filters); and, if possible, designation of CIE coordinates of the same elements.[10] Further, definition of color temperature of the source and a logical scheme for replacement of aged light sources has been recommended above. For color testing it is preferable to use nearly monochromatic stimuli as this greatly simplifies calibration requirements. Similarly (and particularly when non-monochromatic light stimuli are used) the use of light sources which emit continuous spectra simplifies analysis of stimuli.

10. Other Factors

A. Attention signal and shutter noise
In many applications of perimetry it is useful to provide a signal or cue to indicate that a stimulus is about to be presented. Such cues are often auditory. This clearly influences the probability of response and in certain situations may be more effective. Similarly, for long duration stimuli, the noise of an activated shutter can serve the same purpose.

B. Distractions to be avoided
It is recommended that the perimeter be placed in a quiet room where light conditions can be completely controlled, and distractions can be avoided.

C. Relative and absolute scotomas
It is important to differentiate between relative and absolute scotomas. A relative scotomas is defined as a partial visual deficit in a given area of visual field. An absolute scotoma implies total loss of vision in a given field area. Practically, absolute scotomas are usually defined in terms of the largest, most intense target available to the perimetrist. In fact, some response may yet remain and may have been revealed if still larger or more intense targest had been used (assuming stray light effects have been con-

[10] It should be recognized that CIE coordinates as specified for central vision may not be valid for peripheral field test points.

sidered). Thus, it is desirable, in discussions of absolute scotomas, to specify the largest and most intense stimulus employed.

11. Acceptance and Revision of these Standards

a. The proposed standards have been approved by the R.G. on Standards and the Board of the IPS.
b. These Standards, once approved, will remain in force until revised by the R.G. on Standards of the IPS. These Standards must be reviewed every four years and either reaffirmed, modified, or replaced.
c. The R.G. on Standards stands ready to provide reasonable advice, and to offer clarifications relative to matters contained in this set of standards. All correspondence relative to such matters and suggested improvements should be directed to the Secretary of the IPS.

PERIMETRIC GLOSSARY

Committee: Guy VERRIEST (Belgium, *editor),* and (alphabetically) Elfriede AULHORN (GFR), Max EISFELD (GFR), Jay M. ENOCH (USA., chairman of the IPS R.G. on Standards), Franz FANKHAUSER (Switzerland), Lars FRISEN (Sweden), Erik GREVE (The Netherlands, secretary of the IPS), Alberto ISRAEL (Argentina), W. Anna LASZCZYK (Poland), Romuald LAKOWSKI (Canada), Mario MAIONE (Italy), Marion MARRE (GDR), Harutake MATSUO (Japan), Chris PASHLEY (UK), Olga SHCHERBATOVA (USSR) and Virgilio VICTORIA-TRONCOSO (Belgium).

During the preparation of the First International Visual Field Symposium, one of us (G.V.) was asked by Dubois-Poulsen and by other members of the Organizing Committee of this symposium to prepare, for submission to the Concilium Ophthalmologicum Universale (COU), a list of the terms used in visual field investigation, in four languages, namely English, French, German and Spanish. A first list of terms was written in French by Guy Verriest and was subsequently revised, completed and translated into English by Jay M. Enoch, into German by Elfride Aulhorn and into Spanish by Alberto Israel.

During the First International Visual Field Symposium itself, held in Marseille (France) on May 20-24, 1974, a stenciled draft of this glossary was presented. The intention was to subject it to a public enquiry before transmitting it to the COU; however, as all papers of this symposium, the draft was printed without any control of the Organizing Committee and even without any proof corrections by the authors.[1]

On the other hand, the Marseille symposium led to the foundation of the International Perimetric Society (IPS) and of its several Research Groups. Enoch, chairman of the IPS Research Group on Standards, agreed that Verriest should continue to elaborate a multilingual perimetric glossary.

The actual version is much more complete than the first one as it contains 515 terms (instead of 368) in ten languages (instead of four). The choice of the terms intends to cover not only the physio-pathological aspects but also the technical ones, while the chosen languages are not only the most international ones (English, French, German, Spanish, Russian) but also that of other countries with active perimetric research (Italy, Sweden, The Netherlands and Belgium, Poland, Japan).

This version is the result of extensive teamwork. First, the list of items in English was augmented and corrected principally by Enoch, Franz Fankhauser, Lars Frisén, Harutake Matsuo, Chris Pashley and Verriest, the differences between the United Kingdom (UK) and Unites States (US) terms and spellings having been worked out by Enoch and Pashley.

Subsequently Verriest translated all terms into French and sent an English-French stenciled draft to the other team members.

The translations into German were based on Aulhorn's 1974 list and achieved by Marion Marré, Max Eisfeld and Aulhorn.

The translations into Spanish were made by Israel and Virgilio Vittoria-Troncoso.

The translations into Russian were made by Olga Shcherbatova, from the Helmholtz Institute of Moscow, using instead of the cyrillic characters latin ones following the spelling used in the US.

The translations into Italian were made by Mario Maione and those into Swedish by Frisén. Those into Dutch were made by Erik L. Greve and Verriest.

The translations into Polish were first made by W. Anna Laczczyk with the aid of Eisfeld for what concerns the physiological meanings.[2-5] Then the translations were revised by Romuald Lakowski.

The translations into Japanese were made by Matsuo.[6-12,14]

Verriest coordinated the enterprise and watched that the technical terms in the different languages should be as much as possible in accordance with the actual (3rd) edition of the International Lighting Vocabulary published by the Commission Internationale de l'Eclairage (CIE) in nine languages: French, English, German, Russian (with definitions), Spanish, Italian, Dutch, Polish and Swedish (without definitions).[13] There is also a translation of this vocabulary in Japanese, that was used by Matsuo for checking the terms in this language.[14] Verriest was in contact with Gunnar Tonnquist, R.W.G. Hunt and Jo Ann Kinney, appointed by the CIE for the editing of section 45-25 (Eye and Vision) of the next (4th) edition of the International Lighting Vocabulary, and some IPS terms deviant from the actual CIE ones will probably be included in this new edition of the CIE Vocabulary.

Our English items must be considered as the most secure and official ones, and the IPS reference numbers apply primarily to them. When there are differences between the UK and US spellings the UK spellings are given first.

When this can be useful in perimetry, the terms of quantities and units were provided of recommended symbols chosen by Fankhauser, Pashley and Verriest (when possible the same as in the 3rd Edition of the CIE International Lighting Vocabulary); it is for typographical reasons that these symbols were printed only after the English items.

An alphabetical list of the english items was added to make it easier for the reader to find the symbols and the translations from English into the other languages.

It was felt by most team- and IPS RG on Standards members that definitions should be beneficial, at least for some items, but it was decided during the 2nd IPS Symposium held in Tübingen in september 1976 to publish the glossary in its actual form.

At the end of 1976, the Glossary was offered to the Concilium Ophthalmologicum Universale. This organization has the autority to standardize terms, methods of examination, quantities; units *etc.* used in ophthalmology.

However our main purpose is not an attempt to standardize terms. That is best achieved by providing suitable definitions. Rather, we are trying to achieve more effective international understanding in the use of terms and to aid in the development of perimetric research.

REFERENCES

1. Verriest, G., E. Aulhorn, J.M. Enoch & A. Israel. An attempt at standardization of the terminology used in visual field investigation. *Ann. thérap. clin. Ophthal.* 25: 376-390 (1974).
2. *Słownik Terminów Fizycznych*. PWN, Warszawa (1961).
3. *Słownik Techniczny*. 2nd ed., WNT, Warszawa (1969).
4. Adler, F.H. Fizjologia oka. PZWL, Warszawa (1968).
5. Wawrzyniak, M. Polskie mianownictwo histologiczne. PZWL, Warszawa (1968).
6. Draft of lighting section for revised edition of "Japanese scientific terms, Electrical engineering". *J. ill. Engrng Inst. Japan* 55: 514 (1971).
7. Kubota *et al.* Handbook of Optical Technology. Asakura Shoten, Tokyo (1975).
8. Yonezawa, S. *Electronics Dictionary*. Shishjin-sho-kan, Tokyo (1961).
9. *Handbook of Color Science* edited by The Color Science Association of Japan. Nankodo, Tokyo (1962).
10. *Physiological Optics* edited by the Japanese Society of Applied Physics. Asakura Shoten, Tokyo (1975).

11. *Terminology of Physiology* edited by the Japanese Society of Physiology. Igaku-shoin, Tokyo (1972).

12. *Japan Medical Terminology* edited by the Japanese Association of Medical Sciences, Committee on Medical Terminology. Nanzando, Tokyo (1975).

13. *International Lighting Vocabulary,* 3rd ed. common to the CIE and IEC, CIE publ. No 17 (E-1.1). Bureau Central de la CIE, Paris (1970).

14. *International Lighting Vocabulary,* 3rd ed., CIE publ. No. 17 (E.1.1), 1970. Translated into japanese by the Japanese Committee on Illumination (1970).

15. Lauber, H., H.M. Traquair & L.C. Peter. Standardisation of perimetry. XIII. Conc. Ophthal. 1929, Hollandia, Reports. IJdo, Leiden (1929).

IPS	*English*	*Français*
A0	**Stimulation**	**Stimulation**
A1	Inadequate stimulus	Stimulus inadéquat
A2	Adequate stimulus	Stimulus adéquat
A3	Distal stimulus	Stimulus distal
A4	Proximal stimulus	Stimulus proximal
A5	Threshold stimulus	Stimulus liminaire
A6	Subthreshold stimulus	Stimulus subliminaire
A7	Suprathreshold stimulus	Stimulus supraliminaire
A8	Radiation	Rayonnement
A9	Complex radiation	Rayonnement complexe
A10	Monochromatic radiation	Radiation monochromatique
A11	Wavelength - λ	Longueur d'onde
A12	Nanometer - nm	Nanomètre
A13	Spectral distribution	Répartition spectrale
A14	Colour(or)	Couleur
A15	Colour(or) temperature	Température de couleur
A16	Kelvin - K	Kelvin
A17	Dominant wavelength - λ_d	Longueur d'onde dominante
A18	Excitation purity p_e	Pureté d'excitation
A19	Chromaticity coordinates - $x, y; x_{10}, y_{10}$	Coordonnées trichromatiques
A20	Standard illuminant - A, B, C, D_{65}	Illuminant standardisé
A21	Complementary colour (or)s	Couleurs complémentaires
A22	Radiance - L_e	Luminance énergétique
A23	Watt per steradian per square metre(er) - $W.sr^{-1}.m^{-2}$	Watt par stéradian par mètre carré
A24	Luminance-L	Luminance
A25	Candela per square metre(er) - $cd.m^{-2}$	Candéla par mètre carré
A26	Irradiance - E_e	Eclairement énergétique
A27	Watt per square metre (er) - $W.m^{-2}$	Watt par mètre carré
A28	Illuminance - E	Eclairement
A29	Lux - lx	Lux

IPS	*Deutsch*	*Español*
A0	**Reizung**	**Estimulación**
A1	inadaequater Reiz	Estímulo inadecuado
A2	adaequater Reiz	Estímulo adecuado
A3	distaler Reiz	Estímulo distal
A4	proximaler Reiz	Estímulo proximal
A5	Schwellenreiz	Estímulo liminar
A6	unterschwelliger Reiz	Estímulo sub-liminar
A7	überschwelliger Reiz	Estímulo supraliminar
A8	Strahlung	Radiación
A9	zusammengesetzte Strahlung	Radiación compuesta
A10	monochromatische Strahlung	Radiación monocromática
A11	Wellenlänge	Longitud de onda
A12	Nanometer	Nanómetro
A13	spektrale Verteilung	Distribución espectral
A14	Farbe	Color
A15	Farbtemperatur	Temperatura de color
A16	Kelvin	Kelvin
A17	farbtongleiche Wellenlänge	Longitud de onda dominante
A18	spektraler Farbanteil	Pureza de excitación
A19	Farbwertanteile	Coordenadas de cromaticidad
A20	Normlichtart	Iluminante standard
A21	Kompensationsfarben	Colores complementarios
A22	Strahldichte	Radiancia
A23	Watt je Steradiant und je Quatratmeter	Watt por estéreo-radián por metro cuadrado
A24	Leuchtdichte	Luminancia
A25	Candela je Quadratmeter	Candela por metro cuadrado
A26	Bestrahlungsstärke	Irradiancia
A27	Watt je Quadratmeter	Watt por metro cuadrado
A28	Beleuchtungsstärke	Iluminancia
A29	Lux	Lux

IPS	*Russkii*	*Italiano*
A0	**Stimuliatsiia**	**Stimolazione**
A1	Neadekvatnyi stimul	Stimolo inadeguato
A2	Adekvatnyi stimul	Stimolo adeguato
A3	Distal'nyi stimul	Stimolo distale
A4	Proksimal'nyi stimul	Stimolo prossimale
A5	Porogovyi stimul	Stimolo soglia
A6	Podporogovyi stimul	Stimolo subliminare
A7	Nadporogovyi stimul	Stimolo sovraliminare
A8	Izluchenie	Radiazione
A9	Slozhnoe izluchenie	Radiazione complessa
A10	Monokhromaticheskoe izluchenie	Radiazione monocromatica
A11	Dlina volny	Lunghezza d'onda
A12	Nanometr	Nanometro
A13	Spektral'noe raspredelenie	Distribuzione spettrale
A14	Tsvet	Colore
A15	Tsvetovaia temperatura	Temperatura di colore
A16	Kel'vin	Kelvin
A17	Dominiruiushchaia dlina vol-ny	Lunghezza d'onda dominante
A18	Uslovnaia chistota tsveta	Purezza d'eccitazione
A19	Koordinaty tsvetnosti	Coordinate tricomatiche
A20	Standartnyi istochnik izlucheniia	Illuminante standard
A21	Dopolnitel'nye tsveta	Colori complementari
A22	Energeticheskaia iarkost'	Radianza
A23	Vatt na steradian na kvadratnyi metr	Watt per steradiante, per metro quadrato
A24	Iarkost'	Luminanza
A25	Svecha s kvadratnogo metra sv/m^2	Candela per metro quadrato
A26	Obluchennost'	Irradiamento
A27	Vatt na kvadritnyi metr	Watt per metro quadrato
A28	Osveshchennost'	Illuminamento
A29	Liuks	Lux

IPS	*Svenska*	*Nederlands*
A0	**Stimulering**	**Prikkeling**
A1	Inadekvat stimulus	Inadequate prikkel
A2	Adekvat stimulus	Adequate prikkel
A3	Distalt stimulus	Distale prikkel
A4	Proximalt stimulus	Proximale prikkel
A5	Tröskelstimulus	Drempelprikkel
A6	Undertröskligt stimulus	Infraliminaire prikkel
A7	Övertröskligt stimulus	Supraliminaire prikkel
A8	Strålning	Straling
A9	Komplex strålning	Samengestelde straling
A10	Monokromatisk strålning	Monochromatische straling
A11	Våglängd	Golflengte
A12	Nanometer	Nanometer
A13	Spektralfördelningskurva	Spectrale verdeling
A14	Färg	Kleur
A15	Färgtemperatur	Kleurtemperatuur
A16	Kelvin	Kelvin
A17	Dominerande våglängd	Dominerende golflengte
A18	Spektral renhet	Verzadigingsgraad
A19	Kromaticitetskoordinater	Kleurcoördinaten
A20	Standard-ljuskälla	Standaardlichtsoort
A21	Komplementär färg	Complementaire kleuren
A22	Radians	Radiantie
A23	Watt per steradian och kvadratmeter	Watt per steradian en per vierkante meter
A24	Luminans	Luminantie
A25	Candela per kvadratmeter	Candela per vierkante meter
A26	Irradians	Bestralingssterkte
A27	Watt per kvadratmeter	Watt per vierkante meter
A28	Belysningsstyrka	Verlichtingssterkte
A29	Lux	Lux

IPS	*Polski*	*Nihongo*
A0	**Pobudzenie**	**Shigeki**
A1	Bodziec inadekwatny	Futekitō-shigeki
A2	Pobudzenie adekwatne	Tekitō-shigeki
A3	Bodziec obwodowy	En-i-tan-shigeki
A4	Bodziec dosiębny	Kin-i-tan-shigeki
A5	Bodziec progowy	Iki-shigeki
A6	Bodziec podprogowy	Iki-ka-shigeki
A7	Bodziec nadprogowy	Iki-jō-shigeki
A8	Promieniowanie	Hōsha
A9	Promieniowanie kompleksowe	Fukugō hōsha
A10	Promieniowanie monochromatyczne	Tanshokukō
A11	Długość fali	Hachō
A12	Nanometr	Nanometer
A13	Rozkład widmowy	Bunkō-bunpu
A14	Barwa	Iro
A15	Temperatura barwy	Iro-ondo
A16	Kelwin	Zettai-ondo
A17	Długość fali dominująca	Shu-hachō
A18	Czystość pobudzenia	Shigeki-jundo
A19	Współrzędne trójchromatyczne	Shikido-zahyō
A20	Illuminanty normalne	Hyōjun no hikari
A21	Barwy dopełniające	Hoshoku
A22	Luminancja energetyczna	Hōsha-kido
A23	Wat na steradian na metr kwadratowy	Watt per steradian mai hei-hō-meter
A24	Luminancja	Kido
A25	Kandela na metr kwadratowy	l-Heiho-meter shokkō
A26	Natężenie napromienienia	Hōsha-shōdo
A27	Wat na metr kwadratowy	l-Heihō-meter Watt
A28	Natężenie oświetlenia	Shōdo
A29	Luks	Lux

	English	*Français*
A30	Reflection	Réflexion
A31	Specular reflection	Réflexion spéculaire
A32	Diffuse reflection	Réflexion diffuse
A33	Uniform diffuse reflection	Réflexion diffuse orthotrope
A34	Mixed reflection	Réflexion mixte
A35	Regular reflectance - ρ_r	Facteur de réflexion spéculaire
A36	Diffuse reflectance - ρ_d	Facteur de réflexion diffuse
A37	Gloss	Luisance
A38	Transmission	Transmission
A39	Regular transmission	Transmission régulière
A40	Diffuse transmission	Transmission diffuse
A41	Uniform diffuse transmission	Transmission diffuse orthotrope
A42	Mixed transmission	Transmission mixte
A43	Regular transmittance - τ_r	Facteur de transmission régulière
A44	Diffuse transmittance - τ_r	Facteur de transmission diffuse
A45	Absorption	Absorption
A46	Absorptance - α	Facteur d'absorption
A47	Optical density - D	Densité optique
A48	Diffusion	Diffusion
A49	Refraction	Réfraction
A50	Dispersion	Dispersion
A51	Diffraction	Diffraction
A52	Polarized light	Lumière polarisée
A53	Unpolarized light	Lumière non polarisée
A54	Coherent light	Lumière cohérente
A55	Incoherent light	Lumière non cohérente
A56	Temporal modulation	Modulation temporelle
A57	Intermittent stimulation	Stimulation intermittante
A58	Pulsed stimulation	Stimulation pulsée
A59	Periodic pulsed stimulation	Stimulation pulsée périodique
A60	Period	Période

	Deutsch	*Español*
A30	Reflexion	Reflexión
A31	gerichtete Reflexion	Reflexión regular
A32	gestreute Reflexion	Reflexión difusa
A33	vollkommen gestreute Reflexion	Reflexión difusa uniforme
A34	gemischte Reflexion	Reflexión mixta
A35	gerichteter Reflexionsgrad	Reflectancia regular
A36	gestreuter Reflexionsgrad	Reflectancia difusa
A37	Glanz	Brillo
A38	Transmission	Transmisión
A39	gerichtete Transmission	Transmisión
A40	gestreute Transmission	Transmisión difusa
A41	vollkommen gestreute Transmission	Transmisión difusa uniforme
A42	gemischte Transmission	Transmisión mixta
A43	gerichteter Transmissions-grad	Transmitancia regular
A44	gestreuter Transmissions-grad	Transmitancia difusa
A45	Absorption	Absorción
A46	Absorptionsgrad	Absortancia
A47	optische Dichte	Densidad óptica
A48	Streuung	Difusión
A49	Brechung	Refracción
A50	Dispersion	Dispersión
A51	Beugung	Difracción
A52	polarisiertes Licht	Luz polarizada
A53	unpolarisiertes Licht	Luz no polarizada
A54	kohärentes Licht	Luz coherente
A55	inkohärentes Licht	Luz no coherente
A56	zeitliche Modulation	Modulación temporal
A57	unterbrochene Reizung	Estimulación intermitente
A58	pulsierende Reizung	Estimulación pulsada
A59	periodisch pulsierende Reizung	Estimulación pulsada periódica
A60	Periode	Período

	Russkii	*Italiano*
A30	Otrazhenie	Riflessione
A31	Napravlennoe ili zerkal'noe otrazhenie	Riflessione regolare
A32	Diffuznoe otrazhenie	Riflessione diffusa
A33	Ravnomerno-diffuznoe otrazhenie	Riflessione diffusa uniforme
A34	Smeshannoe otrazhenie	Riflessione mista
A35	Koeffitsient napravlennogo otrazheniia	Fattore di riflessione regolare
A36	Koeffitsient rasseiannogo otrazheniia	Fattore di riflessione diffusa
A37	Blesk	Lucentezza
A38	Propuskanie	Trasmissione
A39	Napravlennoe propuskanie	Trasmissione regolare
A40	Rasseiannoe propuskanie	Trasmissione diffusa
A41	Ravnomerno-rasseiannoe propuskanie	Trasmissione diffusa uniforme
A42	Smeshannoe propuskanie	Trasmissione mista
A43	Koeffitsient napravlennogo propuskaniia	Fattore di trasmissione regolare
A44	Koeffitsient rasseiannogo propuskaniia	Fattore di trasmissione diffusa
A45	Pogloshchenie	Assorbimento
A46	Koeffitsient pogloshcheniia	Fattore d'assorbimento
A47	Opticheskaia plotnost'	Densità ottica
A48	Rasseianie	Diffusione
A49	Prelomlenie	Rifrazione
A50	Dispersiia	Dispersione
A51	Difraktsiia	Diffrazione
A52	Poliarizovannyi svet	Luce polarizzata
A53	Nepoliarizovannyi svet	Luce non polarizzata
A54	Kogerentnyi svet	Luce coerente
A55	Nekogerentnyi svet	Luce non coerente
A56	Vremennaia moduliatsiia	Modulazione temporale
A57	Preryvistaia stimulitsiia	Stimolazione intermittente
A58	Pul'siruiushchaia stimuliatsiia	Stimulazione pulsante
A59	Periodicheski pul'-siruiushchaia stimuliatsiia	Stimulazione pulsante periodica
A60	Period	Periode

	Svenska	Nederlands
A30	Reflektion	Reflectie
A31	Spekulär reflektion	Gerichte reflectie
A32	Diffus reflektion	Diffuse reflectie
A33	Uniformt diffus reflektion	Volkomen diffuse reflectie
A34	Blandad reflektion	Gemengde reflectie
A35	Reguljär reflektans	Factor van gerichte reflectie
A36	Diffus reflektans	Factor van diffuse reflectie
A37	Glans	Glans
A38	Transmission	Doorlating
A39	Reguljär transmission	Gerichte doorlating
A40	Diffus transmission	Diffuse doorlating
A41	Uniformt diffus transmission	Volkomen diffuse doorlating
A42	Blandad transmission	Gemengde doorlating
A43	Reguljär transmittans	Factor van gerichte doorlating
A44	Diffus transmittans	Factor van diffuse doorlating
A45	Absorption	Absorptie
A46	Absorbans	Absorptiefactor
A47	Optisk transmissionsdensitet	Optische dichtheid
A48	Diffusion	Verstrooiing
A49	Refraktion	Breking
A50	Dispersion	Kleurschifting
A51	Diffraktion	Buiging
A52	Polariserat ljus	Gepolariseerd licht
A53	Opolariserat ljus	Niet gepolariseerd licht
A54	Koherent ljus	Coherent licht
A55	Inkoherent ljus	Niet coherent licht
A56	Temporal modulering	Temporele modulatie
A57	Intermittent stimulering	Intermitterende prikkeling
A58	Pulserad stimulering	Gepulseerde prikkeling
A59	Periodiskt pulserad stimulering	Periodisch gepulseerde prikkeling
A60	Period	Periode

	Polski	*Nihongo*
A30	Odbicie	Hansha
A31	Odbicie	Kyomen-hansha
A32	Odbicie rozproszone	Kakusan-hansha
A33	Odbicie równomiernie rozproszone	Kintō-kakusan-hansha
A34	Odbicie kierunkowo-rozproszone	Kongō-hansha
A35	Współczynnik odbicia regularnego	Sei-hansharitu
A36		Kakusan-hansharitsu
A37	Połysk	Kōtaku
A38	Przepuszczanie	Tōka
A39	Przepuszczanie kierunkowe	Sei-tōka
A40	Przepuszczanie rozproszone	Kakusan-tōka
A41	Przepuszczanie równomiernie rozproszone	Kanzen-kakusan-tōka
A42	Przepuszczanie kierunkowo rozproszone	Kongō-tōka
A43	Współczynnik przepuszczalności regularnej	Sei-tōkaritsu
A44	Współczynnik przepuszczalności rozproszonej	Kakusan-tōkaritsu
A45	Pochłanianie	Kyūshū
A46	Współczynnik pochłaniania	Kyūshū-ritsu
A47	Gęstość optyczna	Nōdo
A48	Rozproszenie	Kakusan
A49	Załamanie	Kussetsu
A50	Dyspersja	Bunsan
A51	Ugięcie	Kaiseki
A52	Światło spolaryzowane	Henkō
A53	Światło niespolaryzowane	Mu-henkō kō
A54	Światło spójne	Coherent kō
A55	Światło niespójne	Incoherent kō
A56	Modulacja czasowa	Jikan-shūhasū
A57	Pobudzenie przerywane	Kanketsu-shigeki
A58	Pobudzenie pulsujące	Palse-shigeki
A59	Pobudzenie okresowo powtarzające się	Shūkisei-parusu-shigeki
A60	Okres	Shūki

	English	*Français*
A61	Frequency - ν	Fréquence
A62	Hertz - Hz	Hertz
A63	Duty cycle, light dark ratio	Rapport lumière-obscurité
A64	Sinusoidally varying stimulation	Stimulation à variation sinusoïdale
A65	Modulation depth	Profondeur de modulation
A66	Spatial modulation	Modulation spatiale
A67	Modulation transfer function - MTF	Fonction de transfert de modulation
A68	Interferometric resolution	Résolution interférométrique
A69	Object, target (= O)	Objet (= O)
A70	Background (= Bd)	Fond (= F)
A71	Surround (= Sd)	Champ périphérique (= C)
A72	(O, Bd, Sd) shape	Forme (de l'O, du F, du C)
A73	round	rond
A74	elliptical	elliptique
A75	square	carré
A76	(O, Bd, Sd) contour	contour (de l'O, du F, du C)
A77	Edge gradient	Gradient du bord
A78	(O, Bd, Sd) distance -l	Distance (de l'O, du F, du C)
A79	(O, Bd, Sd) diameter -d	Diamètre (de l'O, du F, du C)
A80	Millimetre(er) - mm	Millimètre
A81	(O, Bd, Sd) visual angle - θ	Diamètre angulaire (de l'O, du F, du C)
A82	Minute of arc — $'$	Minute d'arc
A83	Second of arc — $''$	Seconde d'arc
A84	(O, Bd, Sd) area -S	Surface (de l'O, du F, du C)
A85	Square millimetre(er) -mm^2	Millimètre carré
A86	(O, Bd, Sd) solid angle - ω	Surface angulaire (de l'O, du F, du C)
A87	Steradian -sr	Stéradian
A88	(O, Bd, Sd) luminance — L	Luminance (de l'O, du F, du C)
A89	Decibel — dB	Décibel

	Deutsch	*Español*
A61	Frequenz	Frecuencia
A62	Hertz	Hertz
A63	An-Aus-Verhältnis	Duty cycle, relación luz oscuridad
A64	sinusförmige Reizung	Estimulación a variación sinusoidal
A65	Modulationstiefe	Profundidad de modulación
A66	räumliche Modulation	Modulación espacial
A67	Modulationsübertragungs-function	Función de transferencia de modulación
A68	interferometrisches Auf-lösungsvermögen	Resolución interferométrica
A69	Prüfreiz, Prüfobjekt (= P)	Objeto (= O)
A70	Hintergrund (= H)	Fondo (= F)
A71	Umfeld (= U)	Campo periférico (= C)
A72	Form (P, H, U)	Forma (del O, F, C)
A73	rund	redondo
A74	elliptisch	elíptico
A75	quadratisch	cuadrado
A76	Umriss (P, H, U)	Contorno (del O, F, C)
A77	Randgefälle	Gradiente de borde
A78	Abstand (P, H, U)	Distancia (del O, F, C)
A79	Durchmesser (P, H, U)	Diámetro (del O, F, C)
A80	Millimeter	Milímetro
A81	Sehwinkel (P, H, U)	Angulo visual (del O, F, C)
A82	Bogenminute	Minuto de arco
A83	Bogensekunde	Segundo de arco
A84	Fläche (P,H, U)	Superficie (del O, F, C)
A85	Quadratmillimeter	Milímetro cuadrado
A86	Raumwinkel (P, H, U)	Angulo esférico (del O, F, C)
A87	Steradiant	Estéreo-radián
A88	Leuchtdichte (P, H, U)	Luminancia (del O, F, C)
A89	Dezibel	Decibel

	Russkii	*Italiano*
A61	Chastota	Frequenza
A62	Gerts	Hertz
A63	Rabochii tsikl, otnoshenie svet/temnota	Rapporto luce-scuro
A64	Sinusoidal'no izmeniaiushchaiasia stimuliatsii	Stimolazione sinusoidale
A65	Glubina moduliatsii	Profondità di modulazione
A66	Prostranstvennaia moduliatsiia	Modulazione spaziale
A67	Peredatochnaia funktsiia moduliatsii	Funzione di trasferimento della modulazione
A68	Interferometricheskoe razreshenie	Risoluzione interferometrica
A69	Ob"ekt (= O)	Oggetto (= O)
A70	Fon (= F)	Sfondo (= S)
A71	Fonovoe okruzhenie ob"ekta (= Fo)	Campo periferico (= C)
A72	Forma (O, F, Fo)	Forma (dell'O, dello S, del C)
A73	kruglyi	rotondo
A74	ellipticheskii	ellittico
A75	kvadratnyi	quadrato
A76	Kontur (O, F, Fo)	Contorno (dell' O, dello S, del C)
A77	Kraevoi gradient	Gradiente del bordo
A78	Rasstoianie (O, F, Fo)	Distanza (dell' O, dello S, del C)
A79	Diametr (O, F, Fo)	Diametro (dell' O, dello S, del C)
A80	Millimetr	Millimetro
A81	Ugol zreniia (O, F, Fo)	Diametro angolare (dell' O, dello S, del C)
A82	Uglovaia minuta	Minuto d'arco
A83	Uglovaia sekunda	Secondo d'arco
A84	Ploshchad' (O, F, Fo)	Superficie (dell' O, dello S, del C)
A85	Kvadratnyi millimetr	Millimetro quadrato
A86	Telesnyi ugol (prostranstvennyi ugol) (O, F, Fo)	Superficie angolare (dell' O, della S, del C)
A87	Steradian	Steradiante
A88	Iarkost' (O, F, Fo)	Luminanza (dell' O, della S, del C)
A89	Detsibel	Decibel

	Svenska	*Nederlands*
A61	Frekvens	Frequentie
A62	Hertz	Hertz
A63	Arbetscykel, ljus/mörker-kvot	Duty cycle
A64	Sinusoidalt varierande stimulering	Sinusvormige prikkeling
A65	Modulationsdjup	Modulatiediepte
A66	Spatiell modulering	Spatiële modulatie
A67	Överföringsfunktion	Modulatieoverdrachtsfunctie
A68	Interferometrisk resolution	Interferometrische resolutie
A69	Objekt (= O)	Object (= O)
A70	Bakgrund (= Bd)	Achtergrond (= A)
A71	Omgivning (= Og)	Omgevingsveld (= Om)
A72	Form (O, Bd, Og)	(O-, A-, Om-) vorm
A73	rund	rond
A74	elliptisk	elliptisch
A75	kvadratisk	vierkant
A76	Kontur (O, Bd, Og)	(O-, A-, Om-) omtrek
A77	Kant-gradient	Randgradiënt
A78	Avstånd (O, Bd, Og)	(O-, A-, Om-) afstand
A79	Diameter (O, Bd, Og)	(O-, A-, Om-) diameter
A80	Millimeter	Millimeter
A81	Synvinkel (O, Bd, Og)	(O-, A-, Om-) hoekdiameter
A82	Bågminut	Boogminuut
A83	Bågsekund	Boogseconde
A84	Yta (O, Bd, Og)	(O-, A-, Om-) oppervlakte
A85	Kvadratmillimeter	Vierkante millimeter
A86	Rymdvinkel (O, Bd, Og)	(O-, A-, Om-) hoekoppervlakte
A87	Steradian	Steradian
A88	Luminans (O, Bd, Og)	(O-, A-, Om-) luminantie
A89	Decibel	Decibel

	Polski	*Nihongo*
A61	Częstotliwość	Hindo
A62	Herc	Hertz
A63	Funkcja cykliczna	Duty cycle, Mei-an hi
A64	Pobudzenie w postaci sinussoidalnej	Seigen-ha-shigeki
A65	Głębia modulacji	Henchō-do
A66	Modulacja przestrzenna	Kūkanshūhasū
A67	Czynność przekazywania modulacji	Kūkanshūhasū-tokusei
A68	Rozkład interferometryczny	Kanshō-kei kaizōdo
A69	Obiekt (= O)	Shi-hyō (= 1)
A70	Tło (T)	Haikei (= 2)
A71	Tło znaku testowego (TZ)	Shū-i (= 3)
A72	Kształt (O, T, TZ)	Katachi (1, 2, 3)
A73	okrągły	Enkei-no
A74	owalny	Da-enkei-no
A75	kwadratowy	Shikaku, Hō-kei
A76	Kontur /Zarys/ (O, T, TZ)	Rinkaku (1, 2, 3)
A77	Gradient brzeżny	Kido-kōbai
A78	Odstęp (O, T, TZ)	Kyori (1, 2, 3)
A79	Średnica (O, T, TZ)	Chokkei (1, 2, 3)
A80	Milimetr	Mirimētā
A81	Kąt widzenia (O, T, TZ)	Shikaku (1, 2, 3)
A82	Minuta na łuku perymetru	Fun
A83	Sekunda na łuku perymetru	Byō
A84	Powierzchnia (O, T, TZ)	Menseki (1, 2, 3)
A85	Milimetr kwadratowy	Heihō-mirimētā
A86	Kąt bryłowy (O, T, TZ)	Rittaikaku (1, 2, 3)
A87	Steradian	Steradian
A88	Luminacja, jaskrawość świetlna (O, T, TZ)	Kido (1, 2, 3)
A89	Decybel	Decibel

	English	*Français*
A90	(O) intensity – I	Intensité (de l'O)
A91	Candela – cd	Candéla
A92	(O, Bd, Sd) colour(or)	Couleur (de l'O, du F, du C)
A93	red	rouge
A94	orange	orangé
A95	yellow	jaune
A96	green	vert
A97	blue	bleu
A98	violet	violet
A99	purple	pourpre
A100	white	blanc
A101	grey	gris
A102	black	noir
A103	(O, Bd, Sd) Munsell notation	Notation Munsell (de l'O, du F, du C)
A104	(O, Bd, Sd) exposure duration – t	Durée d'exposition (de l'O, du F, du C)
A105	Second of time -s	Seconde de temps
A106	(O) angular velocity	Vitesse angulaire (de l'O)
A107	Degree per second	Degré par seconde
A108	Rate of increase of (O, Bd, Sd) luminance	Vitesse d'augmentation de la luminance (de l'O, du F, du C)
A109	(Photometric) luminance contrast – $C = \Delta L/L$	Contraste (photométrique) de luminance
A110	Corneal illuminance -E_{cor}	Eclairement cornéen
A111	Luminance measured from the position of the centre(er) of the entrance pupil –L_{pup}	Luminance mesurée à la position du centre de pupille d'entrée
A112	Pupil diameter – d_{pup}	Diamètre pupillaire
A113	Pupil area – S_{pup}	Surface pupillaire
A114	Retinal illuminance - E_{ret}	Eclairement rétinien
A115	Troland - td	Troland
A116	Reduced troland - td_r	Troland réduit
A117	Blur of the retinal image	Flou de l'image rétinienne
A118	Intraocular stray light	Lumière diffusée intraoculaire

	Deutsch	*Español*
A90	Lichtstärke (P), Intensität	Intensidad (del O)
A91	Candela	Candela
A92	Farbe	Color (del O, F, C)
A93	rot	rojo
A94	orange	anaranjado
A95	gelb	amarillo
A96	grün	verde
A97	blau	azul
A98	violett	violeta
A99	purpur	púrpura
A100	weiss	blanco
A101	grau	gris
A102	schwarz	negro
A103	Munsell-Bezeichnung (P, H, U)	Notación Munsell (del O, F, C)
A104	Darbietungszeit (P, H, U)	Tiempo de exposición (del O, F, C)
A105	(Zeit-)Sekunde	Segundo de tiempo
A106	Winkelgeschwindigkeit (P)	Velocidad angular (del O)
A107	Grad je Sekunde	Grado por segundo
A108	Geschwindigkeit des Leuchtdichteanstieges (P, H, U)	Velocidad de aumento de la luminancia (del O, F, C)
A109	photometrischer Leuchtdichtekontrast	Contraste (fotométrico) de luminancia
A110	Hornhautbeleuchtungsstärke	Iluminancia corneal
A111	Leuchtdichte gemessen in der Mitte der Eintrittspupille	Luminancia medida en la posición del centro de la pupila de entrada
A112	Pupillendurchmesser	Diámetro pupilar
A113	Pupillenfläche	Superficie pupilar
A114	Netzhautbeleuchtungsstärke	Iluminancia retinal
A115	Troland	Troland
A116	reduziertes Troland	Troland reducido
A117	Unschärfe des Netzhautbildes	Flou de la imágen retinal
A118	intraokulares Streulicht	Luz difundida intraocular

	Russkii	*Italiano*
A90	Intensivnost' (O)	Intensità (dell' O)
A91	Svecha, kandela	Candela
A92	Tsvet (O, F, Fo)	Colore (dell' O, della S, del C)
A93	krasnyi	rosso
A94	oranzhevyi	arancio
A95	zheltyi	giallo
A96	zelenyi	verde
A97	sinii	blu
A98	fioletovyi	viola
A99	purpurnyi	porpora
A100	belyi	bianco
A101	seryi	grigio
A102	chernyi	nero
A103	Oboznachenie po Menzelu (O, F, Fo)	Notazione di Munsell (dell' O, dello S, del C)
A104	Vremia ekspozitsii (O, F, Fo)	Durata di esposizione (dell' O, della S, del C)
A105	Sekunda vremeni	Secondo di tempo
A106	Uglovaia skorost' (O)	Velocità angolare (dell' O)
A107	Gradus v sekundu	Gradi per secondo
A108	Skorost' povysheniia iarkosti (O, F, Fo)	Velocità d'incremento della luminanza (dell' O, della S, del C)
A109	Kontrast iarkosti (fotometricheskii)	Contrasto fotometrico di luminanza
A110	Osveshchennost' na urovne rogovitsy	Illuminamento corneale
A111	Iarkost' izmerennaia iz pozitsii tsentra zrachka	Luminanza misurata dalla posizione del centro della pupilla d'entrata
A112	Diametr zrachka	Diametro pupillare
A113	Ploshchad' zrachka	Superficie pupillare
A114	Osveshchennost' setchatki	Illuminamento retinico
A115	Troland	Troland
A116	Redutsirovannyi troland	Troland ridotto
A117	Nechetkost' (razmytost') izobrazheniia na setchatke	Sfocamento dell'immagine retinica
A118	Rasseiannyi svet vnutri glaza	Luce diffusa intraculare

	Svenska	*Nederlands*
A90	Intensitet (O)	(O-) intensiteit
A91	Candela	Candela
A92	Färg (O, Bd, Og)	(O-, A-, Om-) kleur
A93	röd	rood
A94	orange	oranje
A95	gul	geel
A96	grön	groen
A97	blå	blauw
A98	violett	violet
A99	purpur	purper
A100	vit	wit
A101	grå	grijs
A102	svart	zwart
A103	Munsell-beteckning (O, Bd, Og)	(O-, A-, Om-) Munsellnotatie
A104	Exponeringstid (O, Bd, Og)	(O-, A-, Om-) aanbiedingsduur
A105	Sekund	Tijdseconde
A106	Vinkelhastighet (O)	(O-) hoeksnelheid
A107	Grad per sekund	Graad per seconde
A108	Luminansstegringshastighet (O, Bd, Og)	Snelheid van de vermeerdering van de (O-, A-, Om-) luminantie
A109	(Fotometrisk) luminanskontrast	(Fotometrisch) luminantiecontrast
A110	Corneal belysningsstyrka	Hoornvliesverlichting
A111	Luminans mätt från ingångspupillens centrum	Luminantie gemeten ter hoogte van het midden van de ingangspupil
A112	Pupilldiameter	Pupildiameter
A113	Pupillyta	Pupiloppervlakte
A114	Retinal belysningsstyrka	Netvliesverlichting
A115	Troland	Troland
A116	Reducerad troland	Gereduceerde troland
A117	Oskärpa i retinalbilden	Onscherpte van het netvliesbeeld
A118	Intraokulärt ströljus	Intracular strooilicht

	Polski	*Nihongo*
A90	Światłość (O)	Kyōdo (1)
A91	Kandela	Kandera
A92	Barwa (O, T, TZ)	I-ro (1, 2, 3)
A93	czerwony	Aka
A94	pomarańczowy	Ki-aka (Daidai)
A95	żółty	Ki-i
A96	zielony	Midori
A97	niebieski	A-o
A98	fioletowy	Ki-n
A99	purpurowy	Murasaki
A100	biały	Shiro
A101	szary	Nezumi
A102	czarny	Kuro
A103	Właściwość Munsella (O, T, TZ)	Manseru-Hyōshoku-kei (1, 2, 3)
A104	Okres ekspozycji (O, T, TZ)	Roshutsu-jikan (1, 2, 3)
A105	Sekunda czasu	Dai-niji-sōin
A106	Prędkość kątowa (O)	Kaku-sokudo (1)
A107	Stopień na sekundę	Mai-byo kakudo
A108	Szybkość wzrastania jaskrawości światła (O, T, TZ)	Kido-zōkaritsu (1, 2, 3)
A109	Kontrast jaskrawości światła (fotometryczny)	Kido-taihi
A110	Natężenie oświetlenia rogówki	Kakumaku shōdo
A111	Jaskrawość światła mierzona w środku źrenicy wejściowej	Dōkō -men-kido
A112	Średnica źrenicy	Dōkō kei
A113	Powierzchnia źrenicy	Dōkō ryō
A114	Natężenie oświetlenia siatkówki	Mōmaku shōdo
A115	Troland	Troland
A116	Troland zredukowany	Yūko troland
A117	Zamazanie obrazu siatkówkowego	Momaku zō no boke
A118	Światło rozproszone wewnątrz oka	Gannai-kakusankō

	English	*Français*
A119	Equivalent veiling luminance	Luminance équivalente de voile
B0	**Perception**	**Perception**
B1	Brightness	Phanie
B2	Lightness	Leucie
B3	Hue	Tonalité
B4	Saturation	Saturation
B5	Chromaticity	Chromaticité
B6	Bezold-Brücke phenomenon	Phénomène de Bezold-Brücke
B7	Flicker	Papillotement
B8	Stroboscopic effect	Effet stroboscopique
B9	Speed of perception	Vitesse de perception
B10	Subjective colour(or)s	Couleurs subjectives
B11	Fusion frequency - FF	Fréquence de fusion
B12	Local adaptation	Adaptation locale
B13	Discomfort glare	Eblouissement gênant
B14	Disability glare	Eblouissement perturbateur
B15	Adaptation	Adaptation
B16	Photopic vision	Vision photopique
B17	Mesopic vision	Vision mésopique
B18	Scotopic vision	Vision scotopique
B19	Adaptation curve	Courbe d'adaptation
B20	Break (in adaptation curve)	Point anguleux (de la courbe d'adaptation)
B21	Chromatic adaptation	Adaptation chromatique
B22	Threshold	Seuil
B23	Sensitivity	Sensibilité
B24	Absolute threshold	Seuil absolu
B25	Absolute sensitivity	Sensibilité absolue
B26	Difference (or increment) threshold - ΔL	Seuil différentiel
B27	Difference (or increment) sensitivity — $1/\Delta L$	Sensibilité différentielle

	Deutsch	*Español*
A119	äquivalente Schleierleuchtdichte	Luminancia equivalente al deslumbramiento
B0	**Wahrnehmung**	**Percepción**
B1	Helligkeit	Luminosidad
B2	Helligkeit einer Körperfarbe	Claridad
B3	Farbton	Tono
B4	Sättigung	Saturación
B5	Farbart	Cromaticidad
B6	Bezold-Brücke-Phänomen	Fenómeno de Bezold-Brücke
B7	Flimmern	Flicker, Parpadeo
B8	stroboskopischer Effekt	Efecto estroboscópico
B9	Wahrnehmungsgeschwindigkeit	Velocidad de percepción
B10	subjektive Farben	Colores subjetivos
B11	Verschmelzungsfrequenz	Frecuencia de fusión
B12	Lokaladaptation	Adaptación local
B13	psychologische Blendung	Deslumbramiento molesto
B14	physiologische Blendung	Deslumbramiento perturbador
B15	Adaptationsvorgang	Adaptación
B16	Tagessehen	Visión fotópica
B17	Dämmerungssehen	Visión mesópica
B18	Nachtsehen	Visión escotópica
B19	Adaptationskurve	Curva de adaptación
B20	Kohlrausch-Knick	Punto anguloso (en la curva de adaptación)
B21	Farbumstimmung	Adaptación cromática
B22	Schwelle	Umbral
B23	Empfindlichkeit	Sensibilidad
B24	absolute Schwelle	Umbral absoluto
B25	absolute Empfindlichkeit	Sensibilidad absoluta
B26	Unterschiedsschwelle	Umbral diferencial
B27	Unterschiedsempfindlichkeit	Sensibilidad diferencial

	Russkii	Italiano
A119	Ekvivalentnaia vualiruiu-shchaia iarkost'	Luminanza di velo equivalente
B0	**Vospriiatie**	**Percezione**
B1	Svetlota (sub"ektivnaia iarkost')	Brillanza
B2	Svetlota	Chiarezza
B3	Tsvetovoi ton	Tono di colore
B4	Nasyshchennost' tsveta	Saturazione
B5	Tsvetnost'	Cromaticità
B6	Fenomen Betsol'da - Briukke	Fenomeno di Bezold-Brücke
B7	Mel'kanie	Sfarfallamento
B8	Stroboskopicheskii effect	Effetto stroboscopico
B9	Skorost' vospriiatiia	Velocità di percezione
B10	Sub"ektivnyi tsvet	Colori soggetivi
B11	Sliianie mel'kanii	Frequenza di fusione
B12	Lokal'naia adaptatsiia	Adattamento locale
B13	Diskomfortnaia blestkost'	Abbagliamento intollerabile
B14	Slepiashchaia blestkost'	Abbagliamento disabilitante
B15	Adaptatsia	Adattamento
B16	Fotopicheskoe zrenie	Visione fotopica
B17	Mezopicheskoe zrenie	Visione mesopica
B18	Skotopicheskoe zrenie	Visione scotopica
B19	Krivaia adaptatsii	Curva di adattamento
B20	Perelom krivoi adaptatsii	Spigolo (nella curva di adattamento)
B21	Khromaticheskaia adaptatsiia	Adattamento cromatico
B22	Porog	Soglia
B23	Chuvstvitel'nost'	Sensibilità
B24	Absoliutnyi porog	Soglia assoluta
B25	Absoliutnaia chuvstvitel'-nost'	Sensibitità assoluta
B26	Razlichitel'nyi (inkrement-nyi) porog	Soglia differenziale
B27	Razlichitel'naia (ili inkrementnaia) chuvstvitel'-nost'	Sensibilità differenziale

	Svenska	*Nederlands*
A119	Ekvivalent slöjande luminans	Equivalente sluierluminantie
B0	**Perception**	**Waarneming**
B1	Luminositet	Helderheid
B2	Ljushet	Lichtheid
B3	Färgton	Kleurtoon
B4	Mättnad	Verzadiging
B5	Kromaticitet	Kleursoort
B6	Bezold-Brücke-fenomen	Verschijnsel van Bezold-Brücke
B7	Flimmer	Flikkering
B8	Stroboskopisk effekt	Stroboscopisch effect
B9	Perceptionshastighet	Waarnemingsnelheid
B10	Subjektiv färg	Subjectieve kleuren
B11	Fusionsfrekvens	Versmeltingsfrequentie
B12	Lokaladaptation	Lokale adaptatie
B13	Obehagsbländning	Onbehaaglijke verblinding
B14	Försämringsbländning	Storende verblinding
B15	Adaptation	Adaptatie
B16	Fotopiskt seende	Fotopisch zien
B17	Mesopiskt seende	Mesopisch zien
B18	Skotopiskt seende	Scotopisch zien
B19	Adaptationskurva	Adaptatiecurve
B20	Brott (i adaptationskurva)	Knikpunt (in de adaptatiecurve)
B21	Färgadaptering	Kleuradaptatie
B22	Tröskel	Drempel
B23	Känslighet	Gevoeligheid
B24	Absolut tröskel	Absolute drempel
B25	Absolut känslighet	Absolute gevoeligheid
B26	Differenströskel	Differentiële drempel
B27	Differenskänslighet	Differentiële gevoeligheid

	Polski	*Nihongo*
A119	Luminancjarównoważna zamglenia	Tōkakōmakukido
B0	**Postrzeganie**	**Chikaku**
B1	Jaskrawość	Akarusa
B2	Jasność	Meido
B3	Odcień	Shiki-sō
B4	Nasycenie	Saido
B5	Barwność	Shikido
B6	Zjawisko Bezold-Brücke'a	Bezold-Brücke Genshō
B7	Migotanie	Flicker
B8	Zjawisko stroboskopowe	Stroboscope kōka
B9	Prędkość postrzegania	Chikaku sokudo
B10	Barwy subiektywne	Shukan shoku
B11	Częstotliwość zanikowa	Yūgō-hindo
B12	Adaptacja miejscowa	Kyokusho-junnō
B13	Olśnienie przykre	Fukai-glare
B14	Olśnienie przeszkadzające	Funō-glare
B15	Adaptacja	Junnō
B16	Widzenie fotopowe	Meisho-shi
B17	Widzenie mezopowe	Hakumei-shi
B18	Widzenie skotopowe	Ansho-shi
B19	Krzywa adaptacji	Junnōkyokusen
B20	Załamanie krzywej adaptacji	Kukkyoku ten
B21	Adaptacja chromatyczna	Iro-junnō
B22	Próg	Iki(-chi)
B23	Czułość	Kando
B24	Próg absolutny	Zettai-ikichi
B25	Czułość absolutna	Zettai-kando
B26	Próg różnicy luminacji	Benbetsu-i-ki
B27	Czułość zróżnicowana	Benbetsu-nō

	English	*Français*
B28	Perceived contrast	Contraste perçu
B29	Luminosity contrast	Contraste de luminosité
B30	Colour(or) contrast	Contraste de couleur
B31	Simultaneous contrast	Contraste simultané
B32	Successive contrast	Contraste successif
B33	Contrast threshold (= Weber fraction) – $\Delta L/L$	Seuil de contraste (= fraction de weber)
B34	Contrast sensitivity $L/\Delta L$	Sensibilité au contraste
B35	Modulation threshold – $\Delta L/\Sigma(L_1+L_2)$	Seuil de modulation
B36	Liminal brightness increment (UK) - Just noticeable difference (US)- j.n.d.	Différence à peine perceptible
B37	Visual resolution	Résolution visuelle
B38	Visual acuity	Acuité visuelle
B39	Stereoscopic visual acuity	Acuité visuelle stéréoscopique
B40	Kinetic (= dynamic) visual acuity	Acuité visuelle cinétique (= dynamique)
B41	Achromatic threshold	Seuil achromatique
B42	Chromatic threshold	Seuil chromatique
B43	Photochromatic interval	Intervalle photochromatique
B44	Spatial summation	Sommation spatiale
B45	Successive lateral spatial summation	Sommation spatiale latérale successive
B46	Receptive field	Champ récepteur
B47	Temporal summation	Sommation temporelle
B48	Summation exponent	Exposant de sommation
B49	Summation number	Nombre de sommation
B50	Critical duration	Durée critique
B51	Inhibition	Inhibition
B52	Sensitization	Sensibilisation
B53	Sustained-type visual response	Réponse visuelle de type soutenu
B54	Westheimer function	Fonction de Westheimer
B55	Transient-type visual response	Réponse visuelle de type transitoire

	Deutsch	*Español*
B28	wahrgenommener Kontrast	Contraste percibido
B29	Helligkeitskontrast	Contraste de luminosidad
B30	Farbkontrast	Contraste de color
B31	Simultankontrast	Contraste simultáneo
B32	Sukzessivkontrast	Contraste sucesivo
B33	Kontrastschwelle (= Webers Quotient)	Umbral de contraste (= fracción de Weber)
B34	Unterschiedsempfind-lichkeit	Sensibilidad de contraste
B35	Modulationsschwelle	Umbral de modulación
B36	gerade wahrnehmbarer Unterschied	Diferencia apenas per-ceptible
B37	Auflösungsvermögen des Auges	Resolución visual
B38	Sehschärfe	Agudeza visual
B39	Tiefensehschärfe	Agudeza visual estereo-scópica
B40	Bewegungs-Sehschärfe	Agudeza visual cinética (= dinámica)
B41	achromatische Schwelle	Umbral acromático
B42	chromatische Schwelle	Umbral cromático
B43	photochromatisches Intervall	Intérvalo fotocromático
B44	räumliche Summation	Sumación espacial
B45	räumliche Bewegungssummation	Sumación espacial lateral sucesiva
B46	rezeptives Feld	Campo receptivo
B47	zeitliche Summation	Sumación temporal
B48	Summationsexponent	Exponente de sumación
B49	Summationszahl	Número de sumación
B50	kritische Dauer	Duración crítica
B51	Hemmung	Inhibición
B52	Sensibilisierung	Sensibilisación
B53	stationärer Typ der visuellen Antwort	Respuesta visual de tipo contínuo
B54	Westheimerfunktion	Función de Westheimer
B55	Einschwingtyp der visuellen Antwort	Respuesta visual de tipo transitorio

	Russkii	*Italiano*
B28	Vosprinimaemyi kontrast	Contrasto percepito
B29	Iarkostnyi (svetlotnyi) kontrast	Contrasto di luminosità
B30	Tsvetovoi kontrast	Contrasto cromatico
B31	Odnovremennyi kontrast	Contrasto simultaneo
B32	Posledovatel'nyi kontrast	Contrasto successivo
B33	Porogovyi kontrast (= fraktsiia Vebera)	Soglia del contrasto (= frazione di Weber)
B34	Kontrastnaia chuvstvitel'-nost'	Sensibilità al contrasto
B35	Porog moduliatsii	Soglia di modulazione
B36	Edva zametnoe razlichie	Differenza appena percetibile
B37	Zritel'noe razreshenie	Risoluzione visiva
B38	Ostrota zreniia	Acuità visiva
B39	Stereoskopicheskaia ostrota zreniia	Acuità visiva stereoscopica
B40	Dinamicheskaia ostrota zreniia	Acuità visiva cinetica (= dinamica)
B41	Akhromaticheskii porog	Soglia acromatica
B42	Khromaticheskii porog	Soglia cromatica
B43	Fotokhromaticheskii interval	Intervallo fotocromatico
B44	Prostranstvennaia summatsiia	Sommazione spaziale
B45	Posledovatel'naia lateral'naia prostranst-vennaia summatsiia	Sommazione spaziale laterale successiva
B46	Retseptivnoe pole	Campo recettivo
B47	Vremennaia summatsiia	Sommazione temporale
B48	Pokazatel' summatsii	Esponente di sommazione
B49	Summatsionnoe chislo	Numero di sommazione
B50	Kriticheskaia dlitel'nost'	Durata critica
B51	Tormozhenie	Inibizione
B52	Sensibilizatsiia	Sensibilizzazione
B53	Statsionarnyi tip zritel'noi reaksii	Risposta visiva di tipo sostenuto
B54	Funktsiia Vestkheimèra	Funzione di Westheimer
B55	Neustoichivyi (tranzitornyi) tip reaktsii	Risposta visiva di tipo transitorio

	Svenska	*Nederlands*
B28	Upplevd kontrast	Waargenomen contrast
B29	Luminositetskontrast	Helderheidscontrast
B30	Färgkontrast	Kleurcontrast
B31	Simultankontrast	Simultaan contrast
B32	Successivkontrast	Successief contrast
B33	Kontrasttröskel (= Weber-fraktion)	Contrastdrempel (= fractie van Weber)
B34	Kontrastkänslighet	Contrastgevoeligheid
B35	Modulationströskel	Modulatiedrempel
B36	Nätt (och jämt) märkbar differens	Juist waarneembaar verschil
B37	Upplösning	Visueel oplossend vermogen
B38	Synskärpa	Gezichtsscherpte
B39	Stereoskopisk synskärpa	Stereoscopische gezichtsscherpte
B40	Kinetisk (= dynamisk) synskärpa	Kinetisch (= dynamische) gezichtsscherpte
B41	Akromatisk tröskel	Achromatische drempel
B42	Kromatisk tröskel	Chromatische drempel
B43	Fotokromt intervall	Fotochromatisch interval
B44	Spatiell summation	Spatiële summatie
B45	Successiv lateral spatiell summation	Successieve laterale spatiële summatie
B46	Receptivt fält	Receptief veld
B47	Temporal summation	Temporele summatie
B48	Summationsexponent	Summatie-exponent
B49	Summationstal	Summatiegetal
B50	Kritisk duration	Kritische duur
B51	Inhibition	Inhibitie
B52	Sensibilisering	Sensibilisatie
B53	Sustained-type visual response	Visueel antwoord van het stationair type
B54	Westheimer-funktion	Westheimerfunctie
B55	Transient-type visual response	Visueel antwoord van het transitorisch type

	Polski	*Nihongo*
B28	Kontrast spostrzegalny	Ninshiki-taihi
B29	Kontrast natężenia światła	Meido-taihi
B30	Kontrast barwny	Iro-taihi
B31	Kontrast jednoczesny	Dōji-taihi
B32	Kontrast kolejny	Keiji-taihi
B33	Próg kontrastu (= frakcja Weber'a)	Taihi-shikibetsu-iki (Uēbā-hi)
B34	Czułość kontrastowna	Taihi kando
B35	Próg modulacji	Henchō-iki
B36	Różnica zauważalna	Saishō kachi sa-i
B37	Rozdzielczość wzrokowa	Me no bunkainō
B38	Ostrość wzroku	Shiryoku
B39	Ostrość wzroku stereoskopowa	Rittai shiryoku
B40	Ostrość wzroku kinetyczna (= dynamiczna)	Dōteki shiryoku
B41	Próg achromatyczny	Musaishoku i-kichi
B42	Próg chromatyczny	Yūsaishoku i-kichi
B43	Przedział fotochromatyczny	Ironashi kukan
B44	Sumowanie przestrzenne	Kūkanwa
B45	Sumowanie czasowe i przestrzenne	Keijiteki-sokuhō kūkanwa
B46	Pole odbiorcze	Juyōya
B47	Sumowanie czasowe	Jikanteki kajū
B48	Wykładnik sumowania	Shisū kajū
B49	Liczba kolejna sumowania	Kajū sū
B50	Krytyczny czas trwania	Rikai-jikan
B51	Tłumienie	Yokusei
B52	Sensybilizacja	Kansa (kankō)
B53	Odpowiedź wzrokowa długotrwała	Jikōsei shikaku hannō
B54	Czynność Westheimer'a	Westheimer function
B55	Odpowiedź wzrokowa krótkotrwała	Ikkasei no shikaku hannō

	English	*Français*
B56	Rivalry in the visual field	Rivalité dans le champ visuel
B57	Binocular rivalry	Rivalité binoculaire
B58	Spectral relative luminous efficiency function -$V(\lambda)$	Fonction spectrale d'efficacité lumineuse relative
B59	Purkinje phenomenon	Phénomène de Purkinje
B60	Stiles' π function	Fonction π de Stiles
B61	Directional sensitivity function (= Stiles-Crawford effect)	Fonction de sensibilité directionnelle (= effet de Stiles-Crawford)
B62	Entoptic phenomenon	Phénomène entoptique
B63	Maxwell's spot	Tache de Maxwell
B64	Haidinger's brushes	Houppes de Haidinger
B65	Directional selectivity	Sélectivité directionnelle
B66	Reaction time	Temps de réaction
B67	Optokinetic nystagmus	Nystagmus optocinétique
B68	Attention	Attention
B69	Breadth of attention	Largeur d'attention
B70	Expectancy	Expectation
B71	Conspicuousness	Conspicuité
B72	Distraction	Distraction
B73	Fatigue	Fatigue
B74	Mental processing block	Bloquage mental
B75	Visual performance	Performance visuelle
C0	**Technique**	**Technique**
C1	Psycho-physical method	Méthode psycho-physique
C2	Perimetry	Périmétrie
C3	Campimetry	Campimétrie
C4	Screening method	Méthode de dépistage
C5	Confrontation test	Test de confrontation
C6	Scotometer	Scotomètre
C7	Plate for evaluating scotomas	Carton scotométrique
C8	Tangent screen	Ecran campimétrique (= campimètre)

	Deutsch	Español
B56	Flächenwettstreit	Competencia en el campo visual
B57	Augen-Wettstreit	Competencia binocular
B58	spektrale Hellempfindlichkeitskurve	Funcion espectral de eficacidad luminosa relativa
B59	Purkinjesches Phänomen	Fénómeno de Purkinje
B60	π - Funktion nach Stiles	Función π de Stiles
B61	Stiles-Crawford Effekt	Función de sensibilidad direccional (= efecto de Stiles-Crawford)
B62	entoptisches Phänomen	Fenómeno entópico
B63	Maxwellscher Fleck	Mancha de Maxwell
B64	Haidinger Büschel	Houppes de Haidinger
B65	Richtungsbevorzugung	Selectividad direccional
B66	Reaktionszeit	Tiempo de reacción
B67	optokinetischer Nystagmus	Nistagmus optocinético
B68	Aufmerksamkeit	Atención
B69	Aufmerksamkeitsfeld	Ancho de atención
B70	Erwartung	Expectativa
B71	Auffälligkeit	Conspicuidad
B72	(psychische) Ablenkung	Distracción
B73	Ermüdung	Fatiga
B74	psychologischer Block	Bloqueo mental
B75	Sehvermögen	Performance visual
C0	**Technik**	**Técnica**
C1	psychophysische Methode	Método psico-físico
C2	Perimetrie	Perimetría
C3	Kampimetrie	Campimetría
C4	Screening-Methode	Método de despistaje
C5	Konfrontationstest	Test de confrontación
C6	Skotometer	Escotómetro
C7	skotometrische Testkarte	Cartón escotométrico
C8	Kampimeterschirm	Telón campimétrico

	Russkii	*Italiano*
B56	Sopernichestvo v pole zreniia	Rivalità nel campo visivo
B57	Binokuliarnoe sopernichestvo polei zreniia	Rivalità binoculaire
B58	Spektral'naia krivaia svetovoi chuvstvitel'nosti	Funzione spettrale relativa di visibilità
B59	Fenomen Purkin'e	Fenomeno di Purkinje
B60	π - funktsiia Stailsa	Funzione π di Stiles
B61	Direktsional'naia funktsiia chuvstvitel'nosti (effekt Stailsa - Krauforda)	Funzione di sensibilità direzionale (= effetto di Stiles-Crawford)
B62	Entopticheskii fenomen	Fenomeno entottico
B63	Piatno Maksvella	Macchia di Maxwell
B64	"Shchetki" Gaidingera	Spazzole di Haidinger
B65	Direktsional'naia izbiratel'nost'	Selettività direzionale
B66	Vremia reaktsii	Tempo di reazione
B67	Optokineticheskii nistagm	Nistagmo optocinetico
B68	Vnimanie	Attenzione
B69	Ob"em vnimaniia	Ampiezza d'attenzione
B70	Ozhidanie	Aspettazione
B71	Broskost'	Conspicuità
B72	Otvlechenie vnimaniia	Distrazione
B73	Utomlenie	Fatica
B74	Intellektual'naia blokada	Blocco del processo mentale
B75	Zritel'naia sposobnost'	Prestazione visiva
C0	**Tekhnika**	**Tecnico**
C1	Psikho-fizicheskii metod	Metodo psico-fisico
C2	Perimetriia	Perimetria
C3	Kampimetriia	Campimetria
C4	Skriningovyi metod	Metodo di ricerca
C5	Test sopostavleniia	Test di confronto
C6	Skotometr	Scotometria
C7	Plata dlia otsenki skotomy	Cartone scotometrico
C8	Kampimetricheskii ekran	Schermo campimetrico (= tangente)

	Svenska	*Nederlands*
B56	Rivalitet i synfältet	Rivaliteit in het gezichtsveld
B57	Binokulär rivalitet	Binoculaire rivaliteit
B58	Spectral relative luminous efficiency function	Spectrale ooggevoeligheidscurve
B59	Purkinje-fenomen	Verschijnsel van Purkinje
B60	Stiles-π-funktion	π-functie van Stiles
B61	Direktionell känslighetsfunktion (= Stiles-Crawford-effekt)	Richtingsgevoeligheidsfunctie (= Stiles-Crawford-effect)
B62	Entoptiskt fenomen	Entoptisch fenomeen
B63	Maxwells fläck	Vlek van Maxwell
B64	Haidingers borstar	Haidingerkwastjes
B65	Riktningskänslighet	Directionele selectiviteit
B66	Reaktionstid	Reactietijd
B67	Optokinetisk nystagmus	Optokinetische nystagmus
B68	Uppmärksamhet	Aandacht
B69	Uppmärksamhetsbredd	Aandachtsveld
B70	Förväntan	Verwachting
B71	Tydlighet	Opvallendheid
B72	Distraktion	Afleiding
B73	Trötthet	Vermoeidheid
B74	Mentalt bearbetningsblock	Mentale block
B75	Visuell prestation	Visuële performantie
C0	**Teknik**	**Techniek**
C1	Psykofysisk metod	Psychofysische methode
C2	Perimetri	Perimetrie
C3	Kampimetri	Campimetrie
C4	Screening-metod	Opsporingsmethode
C5	Konfrontationstest	Confrontatietest
C6	Skotometer	Scotometer
C7	Tavla för skotometri	Scotometrische plaat
C8	Kampimeterskärm (= Bjerrumskärm)	Campimeter

	Polski	*Nihongo*
B56	Rywalizacja płaszczyznowa w polu widzenia	Shiya-no-seri-ai
B57	Rywalizacja obuoczna	Ryō-gan-kyōgō
B58	Czynność spektralnego poczucia względnej jasności	Hishikando
B59	Zjawisko Purkinjego	Purkinje genshō
B60	Czynność Stiles'a	Stiles π-function
B61	Czynność siatkówkowego kierunku wrażliwości (= Zjawisko Stiles-Crawford'a)	Stiles-Crawford kōka
B62	Zjawisko entopiczne	Naishi genshō
B63	Plama Maxwell'a	Maxwell han
B64	Miotełki Haidinger'a	Haidinger brushes
B65	Selektywność kierunkowa	Shikōsei-sentakudo
B66	Czas reakcji	Hannō-jikan
B67	Oczopląs wzrokowo-ruchowy	Shisei-ganshin
B68	Uwaga	Chū-i
B69	Zakres uwagi	Chū-i-no-hirogari
B70	Oczekiwanie	Yoki
B71	Właściwość zwracająca uwagę	Kencho
B72	Brak uwagi (psychiczne rozproszenie)	Fuchū-i
B73	Zmęczenie	Hirō
B74	Tłumienie psychiczne	Seishin-teki-block
B75	Postrzeganie wzrokowe	Shi-sagyō
C0	**Określenia techniczne**	**Technique**
C1	Metoda psycho-fizyczna	Shinri-Butsuriteki-hōhō
C2	Perymetria	(Shūhen-)Shiya-sokutei
C3	Kampimetria	(Chūshin-)Shiya-sokutei
C4	Badanie orientacyjne	Screening (Hō)
C5	Test konfrontacyjny	Taimen kensa-hō
C6	Skotometr	Anten-kei
C7	Formularz do pomiaru ubytków perymetrycznych	Anten-hyō
C8	Ekran kampimetryczny	Heimen-shiyakei

	English	*Français*
C9	Angioscotometer	Angioscotomètre
C10	Perimetric arc	Arc périmétrique
C11	Portable hand perimeter	Arc périmétrique portatif
C12	Hemispheric (= cupola, = bowl) perimeter	Périmètre à coupole hémisphérique
C13	Projection perimeter	Périmètre à projection
C14	Monocular perimetry	Périmétrie monoculaire
C15	Binocular perimetry with fusional stimulus	Périmétrie binoculaire avec stimulus de fusion
C16	Participation binocular perimetry	Périmétrie binoculaire de participation
C17	Phase difference haploscopy	Haploscopie par différence de phase
C18	Measurement of peripheral visual acuity	Mesure de l'acuité visuelle périphérique
C19	Werblin's rotating windmill pattern	Moulin tournant de Werblin
C20	Colour(or) perimetry	Périmétrie colorée
C21	Flicker perimetry	Périmétrie de papillotement
C22	Photopic perimetry	Périmétrie photopique
C23	Mesopic perimetry	Périmétrie mésopique
C24	Scotopic perimetry	Périmétrie scotopique
C25	Adaptoperimetry	Adaptopérimétrie
C26	Temporal adaptoperimetry	Adaptopérimétrie temporelle
C27	Steady-state adaptoperimetry	Adaptopérimétrie à état d'adaptation constant
C28	Fundus image-controlled perimetry	Périmétrie sous contrôle du fond d'oeil
C29	Combined method (= check-up)	Méthode combinée (= check-up)
C30	Subjective method	Méthode subjective
C31	Entoptic method	Méthode entoptique
C32	Objective method	Méthode objective
C33	Pupillomotor perimetry	Périmétrie pupillo-motrice

	Deutsch	Español
C9	Angioskotometer	Angio-escotómetro
C10	Perimeterbogen	Arco perimétrico
C11	tragbares Handperimeter	Arco perimétrico portátil
C12	Halbkugelperimeter	Perímetro hemisférico (= de cupula)
C13	Projektionsperimeter	Perímetro de proyección
C14	monokulare Perimetrie	Perimetría monocular
C15	binokulare Perimetrie mit Fusionsreiz	Perimetría binocular con estímulo de fusión
C16	Anteilperimetrie	Perimetría binocular de participación
C17	Phasendifferenz-Haploskopie	Haploscopía por diferencia de fase
C18	Messung der peripheren Sehschärfe	Medida de la agudeza visual periférica
C19	Windmühlendrehmuster nach Werblin	Molino giratorio de Werblin
C20	Farbperimetrie	Perimetría coloreada
C21	Flimmerperimetrie	Flicker perimetría
C22	photopische Perimetrie	Perimetría fotópica
C23	mesopische Perimetrie	Perimetría mesópica
C24	skotopische Perimetrie	Perimetría escotópica
C25	Adaptoperimetrie	Adapto-perimetría
C26	Untersuchung des Adaptationvoranges an einzelnen Gesichtsfeldstellen	Adapto-perimetría temporal
C27	Perimetrie bei festgelegtem Adaptationszustand	Adapto-perimetría en estado de adaptación constante
C28	Perimetrie unter Sicht des Fundus (Fundusperimetrie)	Perimetría con control de fondo de ojo
C29	kombinierte perimetrische Methode	Método combinado (= check-up)
C30	subjektive Methode	Método subjetivo
C31	entoptische Methode	Método entóptico
C32	objektive Methode	Método objetivo
C33	pupillomotorische Perimetrie	Perimetría pupilomotriz

	Russkii	*Italiano*
C9	Angioskotometr	Angioscotometria
C10	Duga perimetra	Arco perimetrico
C11	Portativnyi ruchnoi perimetr	Arco perimetrico portatile
C12	Polusfericheskii perimetr	Perimetro a cupola emisferica
C13	Proektsionnyi perimetr	Perimetro a proeizione
C14	Monokuliarnaia perimetriia	Perimetria monoculare
C15	Binoculiarnaia perimetriia s preriyvistym slivaiushchimsia stimulom	Perimetria binoculaire con stimolo di fusione
C16	Chastichno binokuliarnaia perimetriia	Perimetria binoculaire di partecipazione
C17	Gaploskopiia so sdvigom faz	Aploscopia in differenza di fase
C18	Izmerenie perifericheskoi ostroty zreniia	Misura dell'acuità visiva periferica
C19	"Vetrianaia mel'nitsa" po Verblinn	Mulino di Werblin
C20	Tsvetovaia perimetriia	Perimetria a colori
C21	Mel'kaiushchaia perimetriia	Perimetria di sfarfallamento
C22	Fotopicheskaia perimetriia	Perimetria fotopica
C23	Mezopicheskaia perimetriia	Perimetria mesopica
C24	Skotopicheskaia perimetriia	Perimetria scotopica
C25	Adaptoperimetriia	Adattoperimetria
C26	Vremennaia adaptoperimetriia	Adattoperimetria temporale
C27	Adaptoperimetriia pri postoiannoi adaptatsii	Adattometria allo stato di adattomento costante
C28	Perimetriia pod kontrolem za glaznym dnom	Perimetria sotto controllo del fondo dell'occhio
C29	Kombinirovannyi metod	Metodo combinato
C30	Sub"ektivnyi metod	Metodo soggettivo
C31	Entopticheskii metod	Metodo entottico
C32	Ob"ektivnyi metod	Metodo oggettivo
C33	Pupillomotornaia perimetriia	Perimetria pupillomotrice

	Svenska	*Nederlands*
C9	Angioskotometer	Angioscotometer
C10	Perimeterbåge	Boogperimeter
C11	Portabel handperimeter	Draagbare handperimeter
C12	Hemisfärisk (= halvkule-) perimeter	Halfbolperimeter
C13	Projektionsperimeter	Projectieperimeter
C14	Monokulär perimetri	Monoculaire perimetrie
C15	Binokulär perimetri med fusionsstimulus	Binoculaire perimetrie met fusieprikkel
C16	Participation binocular perimetry	Binoculaire aandeelperimetrie
C17	Fasdifferenshaploskopi	Fasenverschilhaploscopie
C18	Mätning av perifer synskärpa	Meting van het perifere gezichtsscherpte
C19	Werblins roterande kvarnvingemönster	Draaiende windmolen van Werblin
C20	Färgperimetri	Kleurperimetrie
C21	Flimmerperimetri	Flikkerperimetrie
C22	Fotopisk perimetri	Fotopische perimetrie
C23	Mesopisk perimetri	Mesopische perimetrie
C24	Skotopisk perimetri	Scotopische perimetrie
C25	Adaptoperimetri	Adaptoperimetrie
C26	Temporal adaptoperimetri	Temporele adaptoperimetrie
C27	Steady-state adaptoperimetri	Adaptoperimetrie bij constante adaptatietoestanden
C28	Bildlägeskontrollerad perimetri	Perimetrie met funduscontrole
C29	Kombinerad metod	Gecombineerde methode (= check-up)
C30	Subjektiv metod	Subjectieve methode
C31	Entoptisk metod	Entoptische methode
C32	Objektiv metod	Objectieve methode
C33	Pupillomotorisk perimetri	Pupillomotorische perimetrie

	Polski	*Nihongo*
C9	Angioskotometr	Kekkan-anten-kei
C10	Łuk perymetru	Shiyakei no yumi
C11	Perymetr przenośny, podręczny	Temochi-shiya-kei
C12	Perymetr półkolisty	Hankyūjō-shiyakei
C13	Perymetr rzutnikowy	Tōei-shiyakei
C14	Perymetria jednooczna	Tangan-shiya-sokutei
C15	Perymetria obuoczna z bodźcem fuzyjnym	Yugōshigeki o tomonatta ryōgan shiya-sokutei
C16	Perymetria obuoczna z badaniem udziału poszczególnego oka	Furikkā shiya keisoku
C17	Haploskopia o zróżnicowanych fazach	Phase difference haploscopy
C18	Pomiar obwodowej ostrości wzroku	Shūhen-shiryoku no sokutei
C19	Test obracającego się wiatraka Werblin'a	Werblin's kaiten fūsha pattern
C20	Perymetria dla barw	Iro-shiya-sokutei
C21	Perymetria z wywołaniem fuzji migotania	Flicker-shiya-sokutei
C22	Perymetria fotopowa	Meijunnō-shiya-sokutei
C23	Perymetria mezopowa	Hakumeijunnō-shiya-sokutei
C24	Perymetria skotopowa	Anjunnō-shiya-sokutei
C25	Perymetria adaptacyjna	Anjunnō-shiya-sokutei
C26	Badanie adaptacji w różnych miejscach pola widzenia	Jikanteki-junnō-shiya-sokutei
C27	Perymetria po adaptacji do jaskrawości tła	Ittei junnō ji no shiya sokutei
C28	Perymetria oftalmoskopowa	Gantei-zō-seigyo shiyakei
C29	Metoda połączona	Heiyō hō-hō (check-up)
C30	Metoda subiektywna	Jikakuteki hō-hō
C31	Metoda entoptyczna	(Gan)-naishi-gensho-hō
C32	Metoda obiektywna	Takakuteki-hō-hō
C33	Perymetria z obserwacją ruchów źrenicy	Dōkō-undō ni yoru shiya-sokutei

	English	*Français*
C34	Optokinetic perimetry	Périmétrie optocinétique
C35	ERG (= electroretinographic) perimetry	Périmétrie ERG (= électrorétinographique)
C36	VER (= visual evoked response) perimetry	Périmétrie PEV (= potential évoqué visuel)
C37	EEG (= electroencephalographic) perimetry	Périmétrie EEG (= électro-encéphalographique)
C38	Light source	Source lumineuse
C39	Daylight	Lumière du jour
C40	Incandescent lamp	Lampe à incandescence
C41	Projector lamp	Lampe de projection
C42	Halogen lamp	Lampe à halogénure
C43	Fluorescent lamp	Lampe fluorescente
C44	Electronic flash tube	Lampe à éclats
C45	Light emitting diode	Diode lumineuse
C46	Arc lamp	Lampe à arc
C47	Xenon arc	Arc au xénon
C48	Laser	Laser
C49	Point-source	Source ponctuelle
C50	prefocussed	à filament centré
C51	clear	claire
C52	frosted	dépolie
C53	Filament	Filament
C54	Vacillation	Vacillation
C55	Ageing	Vieillissement
C56	Life of a lamp	Durée de la vie d'une lampe
C57	Light housing	Réceptacle de la source lumineuse
C58	Reflector	Réflecteur
C59	Cut-off	Défilement
C60	Projector	Projecteur
C61	Dimmer	Gradateur
C62	Shutter	Obturateur
C63	Screen	Ecran
C64	Diaphragm	Diaphragme
C65	Ground glass	Verre dépoli

	Deutsch	*Español*
C34	optokinetische Perimetrie	Perimetría optocinética
C35	ERG-Perimetrie (= elektroretinographische Perimetrie)	Perimetría ERG (eléctro-retinográfica)
C36	VER-Perimetrie (= Visual Evoked Response-Perimetrie)	Perimetría PEV (= potencial visual evocado)
C37	EEG-Perimetrie (= elektroenzephalographische Perimetrie)	Perimetría EEG (= eléctro-encéfalo-gráfica)
C38	Lichtquelle	Fuente de luz
C39	Tageslicht	Luz diurna
C40	Glühlampe	Lámpara incandescente
C41	Projektionslampe	Lámpara de proyección
C42	Halogenlampe	Lámpara de halógenos
C43	Leuchtstofflampe	Lámpara fluorescente
C44	Blitzröhre	Lámpara de destello electrónico
C45	Leuchtdiode	Diodo luminoso
C46	Bogenlampe	Lámpara de arco
C47	Xenon-Hochdruck-Lampe	Arco de xenón
C48	Laser	Laser
C49	punktförmige Lichtquelle	Fuente puntual
C50	mit vorzentrierter Wendel	preenfocada
C51	klar	clara
C52	mattiert	deslustrada
C53	Wendel	Filamento
C54	Flackern	Inestabilidad
C55	Alterung	Envejecimiento
C56	Lebensdauer einer Glühlampe	Vida de una lámpara
C57	Lampengehäuse	Receptáculo de la fuente luminosa
C58	Reflektor	Reflector
C59	Abschirmung	Cut-off
C60	Projektor	Proyector
C61	Lichtsteuergerät	Regulador de luz
C62	Verschluss	Obturador
C63	Schirm	Pantalla
C64	Irisblende	Diafrágma
C65	Mattglass	Vidrio opal

	Russkii	*Italiano*
C34	Optokineticheskaia perimetriia	Perimetria ottocinetica
C35	ERG (elektroretinograficheskaia) perimetriia	Perimetria ERG (elettroretinografica)
C36	VPZK (perimetriia metodom vyzvannykh potentsialov zritel'noi kory)	Perimetria PVE (potenziali visivi evocati)
C37	EEG (elektroentsefalograficheskaia) perimetriia	Perimetria EEG (elettroencefalografia)
C38	Istochnik sveta	Sorgente luminosa
C39	Dnevnoi svet	Luce diurna
C40	Lampa nakalivaniia	Lampada ad incandescenza
C41	Proektsionnaia lampa	Lampada per proiezione
C42	Galoidnaia lampa	Lampada ad alogeni
C43	Fliuorestsentnaia lampa	Lampada fluorescente
C44	Elektronnaia lampa-vspyshka	Flash a scarica
C45	Svetodiod	Fotodiodo
C46	Dugovaia lampa	Lampada ad arco
C47	Ksenonovaia lampa	Lampada allo xenon
C48	Lazer	Laser
C49	Tochechnyi istochnik	Sorgente puntiforme
C50	Prefokus-lampa	a filamento centrato
C51	chistyi (iasnyi, prozrachnyi)	chiaro
C52	matovyi	smerigliato
C53	Nit' nakala	Filamento
C54	Kolebanie (neustoichivost')	Fluttuazione
C55	Starenie	Invecchiamento
C56	Vremia zhizni (sluzhby) lampy	Durata di vita di una lampada
C57	Svetopriemnik	Ricettacolo della sorgente luminosa
C58	Reflektor	Riflettore
C59	Ekranirovka	Schermatura
C60	Proektor	Proiettore
C61	Reostat dlia regulirovaniia sveta lampy	Regolatore di luce
C62	Zatvor	Otturatore
C63	Ekran	Schermo
C64	Diafragma	Diaframma
C65	Matovoe steklo	Vetro smerigliato

	Svenska	*Nederlands*
C34	Optokinetisk perimetri	Optokinetische perimetrie
C35	ERG (= elektroretino-grafisk)-perimetri	ERG (= electroretinografische) perimetrie
C36	VER (= visual evoked response)- perimetri	VER (= visual evoked response) perimetrie
C37	EEG (= elektroencefalo-grafisk)- perimetri	EEG (= electro-encefalografische) perimetrie
C38	Ljuskälla	Lichtbron
C39	Dagsljus	Daglicht
C40	Glödlampa	Gloeilamp
C41	Projektionslampa	Projectielamp
C42	Halogenlampa	Halogeenlamp
C43	Lysrör	Fluorescentielamp
C44	Blixtrör	Elektronenflitslamp
C45	Lysdiod	Lichtgevende diode
C46	Bågljuslampa	Booglamp
C47	Xenonbåge	Xenonboog
C48	Laser	Laser
C49	Punktformig ljuskälla	Puntvormige lichtbron
C50	prefokuserad	pre-focus
C51	klar	helder
C52	matterad	gematteerd
C53	Glödtråd	Gloeidraad
C54	Ostadighet	Flakkering
C55	Åldrande	Veroudering
C56	Lampas livstid	Levensduur van een lamp
C57	Lamphus	Ruimte voor de lichtbron
C58	Reflektor	Reflector
C59	Avskärmning	Afscherming
C60	Strålkastare	Schijnwerper
C61	Ljusregulator	Lichtregelaar
C62	Slutare	Sluiter
C63	Skärm	Scherm
C64	Bländare	Diafragma
C65	Mattglas	Matglas

	Polski	*Nihongo*
C34	Perymetria optokinetyczna	Gankyū-undō ni yoru shiya-sokutei
C35	Perymetria elektroretinograficzna	ERG ni yoru shiya keisoku
C36	Perymetria z reakcją korową sprowokowaną światłem	VER ni yoru shiya keisoku
C37	Perymetria z blokadą rytmu alfa w EEG	EEG ni yoru shiya keisoku
C38	Źródło światła	Kōgen
C39	Światło dzienne	Chūkō
C40	Zarówka	Hakunetsu-denkyū
C41	Lampa projektorowa	Tōsha-denkyu
C42	Lampa halogenowa	Halogen lamp
C43	Lampa fluorescencyjna	Keikō lamp
C44	Lampa błyskowa elektroniczna	Denshi senkōkan
C45	Dioda emitujaca światło	Hakkō diode
C46	Lampa łukowa	Arc lamp
C47	Ksenon łukowy	Xenon arc lamp
C48	Laser	Laser
C49	Źródło światła punktowe	Ten kōgen
C50	ześrodkowany	Teishōten
C51	przezroczysty	Tōmei
C52	matowany	Tsuyakeshi
C53	Drut żarnikowy	Filament
C54	Mruganie światła	Hendō
C55	Starzenie	Ageing, Rōka
C56	Trwałość żarówki	Jumyō
C57	Obudowa lampy	Light housing
C58	Reflektor	Hanshaki
C59	Zabezpieczenie parzeciwolśnieniowe	Cut-off
C60	Projektor	Tōshaki
C61	Ściemniacz	Chōkōki
C62	Obturator	Shutter
C63	Ekran	Screen
C64	Przesłona	Shibori
C65	Szwło matowane	Suri-garasu

	English	Français
C66	Opal glass	Verre opale
C67	Mirror	Miroir
C68	Semitransparent mirror	Miroir semi-transparent
C69	Neutral density filter	Filtre neutre
C70	Neutral density wedge	Coin photométrique
C71	Neutral step density filter	Filtre neutre à transmission échelonnée
C72	Luminance scale	Echelle de luminance
C73	Luminance step	Echelon de luminance
C74	Colour(or) filter	Filtre coloré
C75	Complementary filter	Filtre complémentaire
C76	Interference filter	Filtre interférentiel
C77	Heat absorbing filter	Filtre anticalorique
C78	Polarizing filter	Filtre polarisant
C79	Nicol prism	Nicol
C80	Polaroid	Polaroid
C81	transparent	transparent
C82	translucent	translucide
C83	opaque	opaque
C84	Projection obliquity	Obliquité de projection
C85	Zoom magnification system	Agrandisseur zoom
C86	Calibration	Calibrage
C87	Photometric control	Contrôle photométrique
C88	Radiometer	Radiomètre
C89	Spectroradiometer	Spectroradiomètre
C90	Photometer	Photomètre
C91	Spectrophotometer	Spectrophotomètre
C92	Photocell	Cellule photoélectrique
C93	Photomultiplier	Photomultiplicateur
C94	Luminance meter	Luminancemètre
C95	Luxmeter	Luxmètre
C96	Standard of light	Etalon de lumière
C97	Comparison surface	Plage de comparaison
C98	Discolouration (UK), discoloration (US)	Décoloration
C99	Yellowing	Jaunissement
C100	Smudging	Salissement
C101	Ametropia	Amétropie

	Deutsch	*Español*
C66	Trübglas, Opalglas	Espejo
C67	Spiegel	Espejo semitransparente
C68	halbdurchlässiger Spiegel	Filtro neutro
C69	Graufilter	Cuña neutra
C70	Graukeil	Cuña neutra de escalones
C71	Graustufenkeil	
C72	Leuchtdichtenbereich	Escala de luminancia
C73	Leuchtdichtestufe	Escalón de luminancia
C74	Farbfilter	Filtro coloreado
C75	Komplementärfilter	Filtro complementario
C76	Interferenzfilter	Filtro interferencial
C77	Wärmeschutzfilter	Filtro de absorción calórica
C78	Polarisationsfilter	Filtro polariscente
C79	Nicol-Prisma	Prisma de Nicol
C80	Polaroid	Polaroide
C81	durchsichtig	Transparente
C82	durchscheinend	Translúcido
C83	lichtundurchlässig	Opaco
C84	Schrägprojektion	Oblicuidad de proyección
C85	Zoomvergrösserung	Sistema Zoom de magnificación
C86	Eichung	Calibración
C87	photometrische Kontrolle	Control fotométrico
C88	Radiometer	Radiómetro
C89	Spektroradiometer	Espectroradiómetro
C90	Photometer	Fotómetro
C91	Spektralphotometer	Espectrofotómetro
C92	Photozelle	Fotocélula
C93	Photomultiplier, Sekundärelektronenvervielfacher (SEV)	Fotomultiplicador
C94	Leuchtdichtemesser	Nitómetro
C95	Beleuchtungsmesser	Luxómetro
C96	Lichtstärkenormal	Patrón luminoso
C97	Vergleichsfeld	Playa de comparación
C98	Verfärbung	Decoloración
C99	Vergilbung	Amarillento
C100	Verschmutzung	Ensuciarse
C101	Ametropie	Ametropía

	Russkii	*Italiano*
C66	Molochnoe steklo	Vetro opalino
C67	Zerkalo	Specchio
C68	Poluprozrachnoe zerkalo	Specchio semi-trasparente
C69	Neitral'nyi fotofil'tr	Filtro neutro
C70	Neitral'nyi fotoklin	Cuneogrigio
C71	Stupenchatye neitral'nye svetofil'try	Filtro grigio a gradini
C72	Iarkostnaia shkala	Scala di luminanza
C73	Iarkostnaia stupen'	Gradino di luminanza
C74	Tsvetnoi fil'tr	Filtro colorato
C75	Fil'tr dopolnitel'nogo tsveta	Filtro complementare
C76	Interferentsionnyi fil'tr	Filtro interferenziale
C77	Teplopogloshchaiushchii fil'tr	Filtro di calore
C78	Poliarizatsionnyi fil'tr	Filtro polarizzato
C79	Prizma Nikolia	Prisma di Nicol
C80	Poliaroid	Polaroid
C81	prozrachnyi	trasparente
C82	poluprozrachnyi	traslucido
C83	neprozrachnyi	opaco
C84	Naklonnaia proektsiia	Obliquità di proiezione
C85	Elektronno usilivaiush-chaia sistema	Ingranditore Zoom
C86	Kalibrovka	Calibrazione
C87	Fotometricheskii kontrol'	Controllo fotometrico
C88	Radiometr	Radiometro
C89	Spektroradiometr	Spettroradiometro
C90	Fotometr	Fotometro
C91	Spektrofotometr	Spettrofotometro
C92	Fotoelement	Cellula fotoelettrica
C93	Fotoumnozhitel'	Fotomoltiplicatore
C94	Iarkometr	Misuratore di luminanza
C95	Liuksmetr	Luxmetro
C96	Etalon sveta	Luce campione
C97	Pole sravneniia	Campo di paragone
C98	Obestsvechivanie	Decolorazione
C99	Pozheltenie	Ingiallimento
C100	Zagriaznenie	Sporcamento
C101	Ametropiia	Ametropia

	Svenska	Nederlands
C66	Opalglas	Opaalglas
C67	Spegel	Spiegel
C68	Halvtransparent spegel	Halfdoorlatende spiegel
C69	Neutralfilter, gråfilter	Neutrale filter
C70	Gråkil	Neutrale wig
C71	Gråstegkil	Neutrale trapverzwakker
C72	Luminansskala	Luminantiebereik
C73	Luminanssteg	Luminantiestap
C74	Färgfilter	Kleurfilter
C75	Komplementärfilter	Complementaire filter
C76	Interferensfilter	Interferentiële filter
C77	Värmefilter	Warmte-absorberende filter
C78	Polariserande filter	Polarizerende filter
C79	Nicolprisma	Nicol
C80	Polaroid	Polaroïd
C81	transparent	doorzichtig
C82	translucent	doorschijnend
C83	opak	ondoorzichtig
C84	Projektionssnedhet	Projectieschuinte
C85	Zoom-förstoringssystem	Zoomvergroter
C86	Kalibrering	Eiking
C87	Fotometrisk kontroll	Fotometrische controle
C88	Radiometer	Radiometer
C89	Spektroradiometer	Spectroradiometer
C90	Fotometer	Fotometer
C91	Spektrofotometer	Spectrofotometer
C92	Fotoelektrisk mottagare	Fotocel
C93	Fotomultiplikator	Fotomultiplicator
C94	Luminansmätare	Luminantiemeter
C95	Luxmeter	Luxmeter
C96	Ljusstandard	Lichtstandaard
C97	Jämförelseyta	Vergelijkingsveld
C98	Missfärgning	Ontkleuring
C99	Gulnande	Vergeling
C100	Nersmutsning	Vervuiling
C101	Brytningsfel	Ametropie

	Polski	*Nihongo*
C66	Szkło mleczne	Opal-garasu
C67	Lustro	Kagami
C68	Lustro półprzezroczyste	Han tōka-maku
C69	Filtr neutralny	Chūsei-filter
C70	Klin szary	Kōgaku-kusabi
C71	Filtr szary stopniowy	Kōgaku dankai-kusabi
C72	Skala luminancji	Kido-memori
C73	Stopień barwnej luminancji	Kido-dankai
C74	Filtr barwny	Iro-filter
C75	Filtr dopełniający	Hoshoku-filter
C76	Filtr interferencyjny	Kanshō-filter
C77	Filtr podczerwony	Netsu-kūshū-filter
C78	Filtr polaryzujący	Henkō-filter
C79	Pryzmat Nicol'a	Nicol
C80	Polaroid	Polaroid
C81	przezroczysty	Tōmei (-tai)
C82	przeświecający	Hantōmei(-tai)
C83	nieprzezroczysty	Futōmei(-tai)
C84	Projekcja ukośna	Sha-tō-sha
C85	System powiększający o zmiennej ogniskowej	Zoom kakudai system
C86	Skalowanie	Kijun-memori
C87	Kontrola fotometryczna	Sokkō-chōsei
C88	Radiometr	Hōsha-kei
C89	Spektroradiometr	Bunkō-hōshakei
C90	Fotometr	Kōdo-kei
C91	Spektrofotometr	Bunkō-kōdokei
C92	Fotoogniwo	Kōdenchi
C93	Fotopowielacz	Kōdenshi-zōbaikan
C94	Nitomierz	Kidokei
C95	Luksomierz	Shōdokei
C96	Wzorzec światła standartowy	Hikari no hyōjunki
C97	Pole porównawcze	Hikaku-ya
C98	Odbarwienie	Taishoku
C99	Zażółcenie	Ōhen
C100	Przybrudzenie	Yogoreru, Osen
C101	Ametropia	Hi-seishi

	English	*Français*
C102	Empty field myopia	Myopie spatiale
C103	Night myopia	Myopie nocturne
C104	Instrument myopia	Myopie instrumentale
C105	Presbyopia	Presbytie
C106	Cycloplegia	Cycloplégie
C107	Resting point of accommodation	Point de repos de l'accommodation
C108	Optical correction	Correction optique
C109	Spectacles	Lunettes
C110	Correction lens	Verre correcteur
C111	Correction lens holder	Support de verre correcteur
C112	Tinted lens	Verre teinté
C113	Contact lens (hard, soft, flexible, corneal, scleral)	Lentille de contact (dure, souple, flexible, cornéenne, sclérale)
C114	Eikonic lens	Lentille eiconique
C115	Achromatizing lens	Lentille supprimant l'aberration chromatique
C116	Blinking	Clignement
C117	Natural pupil	Pupille naturelle
C118	Pupillometer	Pupillomètre
C119	Artificial pupil	Pupille artificielle
C120	Maxwellian view	Vision maxwellienne
C121	Stabilized retinal image	Image rétinienne stabilisée
C122	Chin rest	Mentonnière
C123	Forehead rest	Appui frontal
C124	Dental bite bar	Empreinte dentaire
C125	Occluder	Obturateur
C126	Fixation device	Procédé de fixation
C127	Fixation control	Contrôle de fixation
C128	Infrared image converter	Convertisseur d'image infra-rouge
C129	Visual fixation control	Contrôle visuel de fixation

	Deutsch	*Español*
C102	Raummyopie	Miopía espacial
C103	Nachtmyopie	Miopía nocturna
C104	Geräte-Myopie	Miopía instrumental
C105	Presbyopie	Presbicia
C106	Zykloplegie	Cicloplegia
C107	Akkommodations-Ruhepunkt	Punto de reposo acomodativo
C108	optische Korrectur	Correción óptica
C109	Brille	Anteojos
C110	Korrekturlinse	Cristal corrector
C111	Korrekturlinsenhalter	Soporte del cristal corrector
C112	getöntes Glas	Cristal coloreado
C113	Kontaktlinse (hart, weich, flexibel, corneal, skleral)	Lente de contacto (duro, blando, flexible, corneal, escleral)
C114	Aniseikonie-Linse	Lente eicónica
C115	Linse zum Ausgleich der chromatischen Aberration des Auges	Lente suprimiendo la aberración cromática
C116	Blinzeln	Parpadeo
C117	natürliche Pupille	Pupila natural
C118	Pupillometer	Pupilómetro
C119	künstliche Pupille	Pupila artificial
C120	Maxwellsche Abbildung	Visión maxweliana
C121	stabilisiertes Netzhautbild	Imágen retiniana estabilizada
C122	Kinnstütze	Mentonera
C123	Stirnstütze	Apoyo frontal
C124	Beissbrettchen	Impresión dental
C125	Verschlussklappe	Obturador
C126	Fixationsvorrichtung	Procedimiento de fijación
C127	Fixationskontrolle	Control de fijación
C128	Infrarot-Bildwandler	Convertidor de imágen infra-rojo
C129	Fixationskontrolle	Control visual de fijación

	Russkii	*Italiano*
C102	Miopiia "pustogo polia"	Miopia spaziale
C103	Nochnaia blizorukost' (miopiia)	Miopia notturna
C104	Instrumental'naia miopiia	Miopia strumentale
C105	Presbiopiia	Presbiopia
C106	Tsikloplegiia	Cicloplegia
C107	Punkt pokoia akkomodatsii	Punto di riposa dell' accomodazione
C108	Opticheskaia korrektsiia	Correzione ottica
C109	Ochki	Occhiali
C110	Korrigiruiushchee steklo	Lente correttiva
C111	Oprava dlia korrigiruiushchego stekla	Supporto di lente correttiva
C112	Linza s izbiratel'nym tsvetopogloshcheniem	Lente colorata
C113	Kontaktnye linzy (tverdye, miagkie, gibkie, rogovichnye, skleral'nye	Lente di contatto (dura, molle, flessibile, corneale, sclerale)
C114	Eikonicheskaia linza	Lente eiconica
C115	Linza, umen'shaiushchaia khromaticheskyiu aberratsiiu	Lente acromatizzante
C116	Miganie	Ammiccamento
C117	Estestvennyi zrachok	Pupilla naturale
C118	Pupillometr	Pupillometro
C119	Iskusstvennyi zrachok	Pupilla artificiale
C120	Maksvellovskii obraz	Visione Maxwelliana
C121	Stabilizirovannoe setchatochnoe izobrazhenie	Immagine retinica stabilizzata
C122	Podborodnik	Mentoniera
C123	Podlobnik	Appoggia fronte
C124	Zuboderzhatel'	Impronta dentaria
C125	Okkliuder	Otturatore
C126	Fiksatsionnoe ustroistvo	Sistema di fissazione
C127	Kontrol' fiksatsii	Controllo della fissazione
C128	Infrakrasnyi preobrazovatel' izobrazheniia	Convertitore d'immagine infrarossa
C129	Zritel'nyi kontrol' fiksatsii	Controllo visivo della fissazione

	Svenska	*Nederlands*
C102	Empty field myopia	Ruimtemyopie
C103	Nattmyopi	Nachtmyopie
C104	Instrumentmyopi	Instrumentmyopie
C105	Presbyopi	Presbyopie
C106	Cykloplegi	Cycloplegie
C107	Ackommodations-vilopunkt	Accommodatierustpunt
C108	Optisk korrektion	Optische correctie
C109	Glasögon	Bril
C110	Korrektionslins	Correctieglas
C111	Korrektionslinshållare	Correctieglashouder
C112	Färgad lins	Gekleurde lens
C113	Kontaktlins (hård, mjuk, flexibel, corneal, scleral)	Contactlens (hard, zacht, plooibaar, corneaal, scleraal)
C114	Eikonisk lins	Eikonische lens
C115	Akromatiserande lins	Lens voor de correctie van de chromatische aberratie
C116	Blinka	Knipperen
C117	Naturlig pupill	Natuurlijke pupil
C118	Pupillometer	Pupillometer
C119	Artificiell pupill	Kunstmatige pupil
C120	Maxwellian view	Maxwelliaans zicht
C121	Stabiliserad näthinnebild	Gestabiliseerd netvliesbeeld
C122	Hakstöd	Kinsteun
C123	Pannstöd	Voorhoofdsteun
C124	Bitbräda	Bijtstuk
C125	Ockluder	Ooglap
C126	Fixationsanordning	Fixatiemethode
C127	Fixationskontroll	Fixatiecontrole
C128	Infraröd bildomvandlare	Apparaat voor het omzetten van een infraroodbeeld
C129	Visuell fixationskontroll	Visuele fixatiecontrole

	Polski	Nihongo
C102	Kūkan-kinshi	Krótkowzroczność przestrzenna
C103	Yakan-kinshi	Krótkowzroczność nocna
C104	Kikai-kinshi	Krótkowzroczność przyrządowa
C105	Rōshi	Starczowzroczność
C106	Mōyōkin-mahi	Cykloplegia
C107	Chōsetsu-ansei-i	Punkt spoczynkowy akomodacji
C108	Kōgakuteki-kyōsei	Korekcja optyczna
C109	Gankyō	Okulary
C110	Kyōsei lens	Szkło korekcyjne
C111	Gankyō-shiken-waku	Oprawka do szkieł próbnych
C112	Iro lens	Szło przyciemnione
C113	Contakuto lens (hādo, sofuto, furekishiburu, kakumaku, kyōmaku)	Szło kontaktowe (twarde, miękkie, elastyczne, rogówkowe, twardówkowe)
C114	Eikonic lens	Soczewka anizeikoniczna
C115	Irokeshi-lens	Soczewka z neutralizacją aberacji chromatycznej
C116	Shunmoku	Mruganie
C117	Shizen-dōkō	Źrenica
C118	Dōkōkei	Źrenicomierz
C119	Jinkō-dōkō	Źrenica sztuczna
C120	Maxwell-shi	Obserwacja Maxwella
C121	Seishi mōmaku zō	Obraz siatkówkowy ustalony
C122	Ago-dai	Wspornik brody
C123	Hitai uke	Wspornik czoła
C124	Kami-ban	Zacisk zębowy
C125	Shagan-shi	Obturator
C126	Koshi sōchi	Urządzenie do badania fiksacji
C127	Koshi no control	Sprawdzanie fiksacji
C128	Sekigai-converter	Aparat przetwarzający obrazy w podczerwieni
C129	Me ni yoru koshi no control	Sprawdzanie wzrokowe fiksacji

	English	*Français*
C130	Electronic fixation monitor	Moniteur électronique de fixation
C131	Isopter perimetry	Périmétrie d'isoptères
C132	Profile perimetry	Périmétrie en profil
C133	Meridional perimetry	Périmétrie méridienne
C134	Circular perimetry	Périmétrie circulaire
C135	Kinetic perimetry	Périmétrie cinétique
C136	centripetal	centripète
C137	centrifugal	centrifuge
C138	clockwise	dans le sens des aiguilles d'une montre
C139	anticlockwise (UK), counter-clockwise (US)	dans le sens contraire à celui des aiguilles d'une montre
C140	Rate of movement	Vitesse de translation
C141	Automatic object translation	Mouvement automatique de l'objet
C142	Static perimetry	Périmétrie statique
C143	Single stimulus	Stimulus unique
C144	Multiple stimuli	Stimuli multiples
C145	Multiple pattern	Pattern multiples
C146	Frequency of presentation	Fréquence de présentation
C147	Flash	Eclair
C148	Tachistoscopic presentation	Présentation tachystoscopique
C149	Kinetic-static perimetry	Périmétrie cinético-statique
C150	Perimetrist	Périmétriste
C151	Subject (= observer, = patient)	Sujet (= observateur, = patient)
C152	experienced	expérimenté
C153	inexperienced	non expérimenté
C154	Ascending method of limits	Méthode ascendante de limites
C155	Descending method of limits	Méthode descendante de limites
C156	Frequency-of-seeing curve	Courbe de fréquence de perception
C157	Forced binary choice	Choix forcé binaire
C158	Forced multiple choice	Choix forcé multiple
C159	Subject's response criterion	Critère personnel de réponse

	Deutsch	*Español*
C130	elektronische Fixationskontrolle	Control electrónico de fijación
C131	Isopterenperimetrie	Perimetría isoptérica
C132	Profilperimetrie	Perimetría de perfil
C133	Perimetrie in Meridianen	Perimetría meridiana
C134	Perimetrie in Kreisbogen	Perimetría circular
C135	kinetische Perimetrie	Perimetría cinética
C136	zentripetal	centrípeto
C137	zentrifugal	centrífugo
C138	im Uhrzeigersinn	en el sentido de las agujas del reloj
C139	gegen dem Uhrzeigersinn	en el sentido contrario a las agujas del reloj
C140	Prüfobjektgeschwindigkeit	Velocidad de translado
C141	automatische Objektbewegung	Movimiento automático del objeto
C142	statische Perimetrie	Perimetría estática
C143	Einzelreiz	Estímulo único
C144	Mehrfachreiz	Estímulos múltiples
C145	Reizmuster	Modelos múltiples
C146	Darbietungsfrequenz	Frecuencia de presentación
C147	Blitz	Flash
C148	tachystokopische Darbietung	Presentación taquistoscópica
C149	statisch-kinetische Perimetrie	Perimetría cinética estática
C150	Perimetrist	Perimetrista
C151	Prüfling (= Beobachter, = Patient)	Sujeto (= observador, = paciente)
C152	geübt	experimentado
C153	ungeübt	no experimentado
C154	Schwellenbestimmung mit ansteigenden Reiz	Método ascendente de límites
C155	Schwellenbestimmung mit absteigenden Reiz	Método descendente de límites
C156	Kurve der Wahrnemungshäufigkeit	Curva de frecuencia de percepción
C157	obligatorische binäre Wahl	Elección forzada binaria
C158	obligatorische Vielfach-Wahl	Elección forzada múltiple
C159	persönliches Antwortkriterium	Criterio personal de respuesta

	Russkii	*Italiano*
C130	Elektronnyi monitor dlia fiksatsii	Controllo elettronico di fissazione
C131	Izopternaia perimetriia	Perimetria d'isoptera
C132	Profil'naia perimetriia	Perimetria di profilo
C133	Meridional'naia perimetriia	Perimetria meridiana
C134	Tsirkuliarnaia perimetriia	Perimetria circolare
C135	Kineticheskaia perimetriia	Perimetria cinetica
C136	tsentrostremitel'nyi	centripeto
C137	tsentrobezhnyi	centrifugo
C138	po chasovoi strelke	nel senso delle lancette dell'orologio
C139	protiv chasovoi strelki	nel senso contrario alle lancette dell'orologio
C140	Skorost' dvizheniia	Velocità di traslazione
C141	Avtomaticheskoe dvizhenie ob"ekta	Movimento automatico della mira
C142	Staticheskaia perimetriia	Perimetria statica
C143	Odinochnyi stimul	Stimolo unico
C144	Mnozhestvennye stimuly	Stimoli multipli
C145	Slozhnyi ob"ekt (pattern)	Configurazioni multiple
C146	Chastota pred"iavleniia	Frequenza di presentazione
C147	Vspyshka	Flash (lampo)
C148	Takhiskopicheskoe pred"iavlenie	Presentazione tachistoscopica
C149	Kinetiko-staticheskaiia perimetriia	Perimetria cinetico-statica
C150	Perimetrist	Perimetrista
C151	Sub"ekt (= nabliudatel', = patsient)	Soggetto (= osservatore, = paziente)
C152	Obsledovannyi	Esperto
C153	neobsledovannyi	inesperto
C154	Metod opredeleniia poroga na ischezisovenie	Metodo ascendente del limite
C155	Metod opredeleniia poroga na poiavlenie	Metodo discendente del limite
C156	Krivaia chastoty videniia	Curva di frequenza di percezione
C157	Prinuditel'nyi binarnyi vybor	Scelta forzata binaria
C158	Prinuditel'nyi vybor iz mnorzhestva	Scelta forzata multipla
C159	Kriterii sub"ektivnogo otveta	Criterio di risposta del soggetto

	Svenska	Nederlands
C130	Elektronisk fixationsmonitor	Electronische fixatiemonitor
C131	Isopterperimetri	Isopterperimetrie
C132	Profilperimetri	Profielperimetrie
C133	Meridianperimetri	Meridiaanperimetrie
C134	Cirkulär perimetri	Circulaire perimetrie
C135	Kinetisk perimetri	Kinetische perimetrie
C136	centripetal	centripetaal
C137	centrifugal	centrifugaal
C138	medurs	met de klok mee
C139	moturs	tegen de klok
C140	Rörelsehastighet	Bewegingsnelheid
C141	Automatisk objektrörelse	Automatische objectbeweging
C142	Statisk perimetri	Statische perimetrie
C143	Enkelt stimulus	Enkelvoudige prikkel
C144	Multipla stimuli	Meervoudige prikkels
C145	Mönster	Meervoudige patronen
C146	Presentationsfrekvens	Aanbiedingsfrequentie
C147	Blixt	Flits
C148	Takistoskopisk presentation	Tachistoscopische aanbieding
C149	Kinetisk-statisk perimetri	Kinetisch-statische perimetrie
C150	Perimetrist	Perimetrist
C151	Försöksperson (= Patient)	Proefpersoon (= waarnemer, = patiënt)
C152	erfaren	ervaren
C153	oerfaren	onervaren
C154	Stigande styrka	Stijgende drempelmethode
C155	Fallande styrka	Dalende drempelmethode
C156	Frequency-of-seeing curve	Frequency-of-seeing curve
C157	Binärt tvångsval	Verplichte binaire keus
C158	Tvångsval vid flervalsprov	Verplichte meervoudige keus
C159	Försökspersons svarskriterium	Persoonlijk antwoordcriterium

	Polski	*Nihongo*
C130	Badanie elektroniczne fiksacji	Denkiteki koshi monitor
C131	Perymetria izopterowa	Isopter perimetry
C132	Perymetria profilowa	Profile perimetry
C133	Perymetria południkowa	Meridian perimetry
C134	Perymetria okrężna	Circular perimetry
C135	Perymetria kinetyczna	Dōteki shiya
C136	dośrodkowy	Kyūshinteki-no
C137	odśrodkowy	Enshinteki-no
C138	w kierunku wskazówek zegara	Tokei no hari to dō-hōkō
C139	przeciwnie do wskazówek zegara	Tokei no hari to hantai hōkō
C140	Szybkość ruchu	Idō-sokudo
C141	Ruch automatyczny obiektu	Jidōteki-shihyo-ido
C142	Perymetria statyczna	Seiteki shiya
C143	Bodziec pojedyńczy	Tansū-shigeki
C144	Bodźce mnogie	Tasū-shigeki
C145	Wzory wielorakie	Multiple pattern
C146	Częstość prezentacji	Teiji no hindo
C147	Błysk	Senkō (flash)
C148	Prezentacja tachytoskopowa	Tachystoscopic presentation
C149	Perymetria kinetyczno-statyczna	Dōteki-seiteki-shiya
C150	Perymetrysta	Perimetrist
C151	Osoba badana (= pacjent)	Hikenja
C152	doświadczony	Keiken no aru
C153	niedoświadczony	Mi-keiken no
C154	Pomiar wzrastającej wartości progowej	Jōsho kyokugen-ho
C155	Pomiar obniżającej się wartości progowej	Kakō kyokugen-ho
C156	Krzywa częstotliwości wzrokowej	Shinin-kyokusen
C157	Przymus do dwojakiego wyboru	Kyōsei-nigen-sentaku
C158	Przymus do wyboru spośród wielu	Kyōsei-takōshiki-sentaku
C159	Kryterium odpowiedzi osoby badanej	Hikenja no hannō kijun

	English	*Français*
C160	Judgement time	Temps de jugement
C161	(Degree of) Cooperation of the subject	(Degré de) Collaboration du sujet
C162	Motivation	Motivation
C163	Reaction time	Temps de réaction
C164	Chronometer	Chronomètre
C165	Test period	Période d'essais
C166	Rest period	Période de repos
C167	Accommodation	Accommodation
C168	Relaxation of accommodation	Décompensation de l'accommodation
C169	Spiral shaped pattern	Tracé en spirale
C170	Star shaped pattern	Tracé en étoile
C171	Repeat static test	Test statique à répétition
C172	Extinction phenomenon	Phénomène d'extinction
C173	False positive response	Réponse faussement positive
C174	False negative response	Réponse faussement négative
C175	Delayed response	Réponse retardée
C176	Signal device	Système de signalisation
C177	Verbal response	Réponse verbale
C178	Manual response	Réponse manuelle
C179	Push-button	Bouton-pressoir
C180	Buzzer	Signal sonore
C181	Manual recording	Enregistrement manuel
C182	Semi-automatic recording	Enregistrement semi-automatique
C183	Automatic recording	Enregistrement automatique
C184	Automation	Automation
C185	Programme (UK), Program (US)	Programme
C186	Computerised perimetry	Périmétrie par ordinateur
C187	Chart	Schéma d'enregistrement
C188	Chart scale	Echelle du schéma
C189	Polygonal connection (of isopter)	Relier les points (d'un isoptère) par des droites

	Deutsch	Español
C160	Beurteilungszeit	Tiempo de decisión
C161	(Grad der) Mitarbeit des Prüflings	(Grado de) Colaboración del sujeto
C162	Motivation	Motivación
C163	Reaktionszeit	Tiempo de reacción
C164	Chronometer	Cronómetro
C165	Untersuchungsdauer	Período de ensayo
C166	Pausendauer	Período de reposo
C167	Akkommodation	Acomodación
C168	Akkommodationsentspannung	Descompensación de la acomodación
C169	spiralförmiges Gesichtsfeld	Trazado en espiral
C170	sternförmiges Gesichtsfeld	Trazado en estrella
C171	Statische Wiederholungsprüfung	Test estático de repetición
C172	Löschphänomen	Fenómeno de extinción
C173	falsch-positive Antwort	Respuesta falsamente positiva
C174	falsch-negative Antwort	Respuesta falsamente negativa
C175	verzögerte Antwort	Respuesta atrasada
C176	Signalvorrichtung	Sistema de señalización
C177	mündliche Antwort	Respuesta verbal
C178	manuelle Antwort	Respuesta manual
C179	Druckknopf	Botón
C180	Summer	Señal sonora
C181	manuelle Aufzeichnung	Registro manual
C182	halbautomatische Registrierung	Registro semi-automático
C183	automatische Registrierung	Registro automático
C184	Automatisierung	Automatización
C185	Programm	Programa
C186	Computer-Perimetrie	Perimetría por computador
C187	(Registrier-)Schema	Esquema de registro
C188	Registrier-Massstab	Escala del esquema de registro
C189	geradlinige Verbindung der Isopterenmesspunkte	Unir los puntos (de una isóptera) por rectas

	Russkii	*Italiano*
C160	Vremia priniatiia resheniia	Tempo di giudizio
C161	(Stepen') kooperatsiia ispytuemogo	(Grado di) Collaborazione del soggetto
C162	Motivatsiia	Motivazione
C163	Vremia reaktsii	Tempo di reazione
C164	Khronometr	Cronometro
C165	Period testirovaniia	Periodo di seduta
C166	Period pokoia	Periodo di riposo
C167	Akkomodatsiia	Accomodazione
C168	Rasslablenie akkomodatsii	Rilasciamento dell'accomodazione
C169	Spiralevidnyi pattern	Tracciato a spirale
C170	Zvezdchatyi pattern	Tracciato stellato
C171	Povtornyi staticheskii test	Test statico a ripetizione
C172	Fenomen ugasaniia	Fenomeno d'estinzione
C173	Oshibochnyi polozhitel'nyi otvet	Risposta falsamente positiva
C174	Oshibochnyi otritsatel'nyi otvet	Risposta falsamente negativa
C175	Pozdnii otvet	Risposta ritardata
C176	Signal'noe ustroistvo	Apparecchio per il segnale
C177	Slovesnyi otvet	Risposta verbale
C178	Otvet rukoi	Risposta manuale
C179	Nazhimnaia knopka	Pulsante
C180	Zummer	Segnale sonoro
C181	Ruchnaia registratsiia	Registrazione manuale
C182	Poluavtomaticheskaia registratsiia	Registrazione semiautomatica
C183	Avtomaticheskaia registratsiia	Registrazione automatica
C184	Avtomatizatsiia	Automazione
C185	Programma	Programma
C186	Comp'iuternaia perimetriia	Perimetria computerizzata
C187	Skhema registratsii	Schema di registrazione
C188	Masshtab skhemy	Scala dello schema
C189	Poligonal'noe soedinenie (izopter)	Connessione poligonale (dell'isottera)

	Svenska	*Nederlands*
C160	Bedömningstid	Beoordelingsduur
C161	Grad av medverkan	(Mate van) Medewerking van de proefpersoon
C162	Motivation	Motivatie
C163	Reaktionstid	Reactietijd
C164	Tidur	Chronometer
C165	Testperiod	Testperiode
C166	Viloperiod	Rustperiode
C167	Ackommodation	Accommodatie
C168	Avslappning av ackommodation	Accommodatiedecompen-satie
C169	Spiralmönster	Spiraalvormig verloop
C170	Stjärnmönster	Stervormig verloop
C171	Upprepat statiskt test	Herhaalde statische proef
C172	Extinktionsfenomen	Extinctiefenomeen
C173	Falskt positivt svar	Vals positief antwoord
C174	Falskt negativt svar	Vals negatief antwoord
C175	Försenat svar	Vertraagd antwoord
C176	Signalanordning	Signalisatiesysteem
C177	Muntligt svar	Mondeling antwoord
C178	Manuellt svar	Manueel antwoord
C179	Tryck-knapp	Drukknop
C180	Summer	Zoemer
C181	Manuell registrering	Manuele registratie
C182	Halvautomatisk registrering	Semi-automatische registra-tie
C183	Automatisk registrering	Automatische registratie
C184	Automatisering	Automatisering
C185	Program	Program
C186	Dator-perimetri	Computerperimetrie
C187	Diagram	Registratieschema
C188	Diagramskala	Registratieschemaschaal
C189	Polygonal isopterkon-struktion	Veelhoekige verbinding van de (isopter)punten

	Polski	*Nihongo*
C160	Czas orzeczenia	Handan-jikan
C161	Stopień współpracy osoby badanej	Hikenja no kyōryoku no doai
C162	Uzasadnienie	Dōkizuke
C163	Czas reakcji	Hanno jikan
C164	Chronometr	Keiji-dokei
C165	Zespół badań	Kensa kikan
C166	Okres odpoczynku	Kyu-shi kikan
C167	Akomodacja	Chōsetsu
C168	Wyłączenie akomodacji	Chōsetsu no shikan
C169	Pole widzenia spiralne	Rasenkei pattern
C170	Pole widzenia w kształcie gwiazdy	Hoshigata pattern
C171	Test statyczny kilkakrotnie powtarzany	Hanpuku seiteki test
C172	Zjawisko	Shō-kyo genshō
C173	Odpowiedź błędna pozytywna	Gi-yōsei-hannō
C174	Odpowiedź błędna negatywna	Gi-insei-hannō
C175	Odpowiedź opóźniona	Chien-hannō
C176	Układ sygnalizacyjny	Shingō-sōchi
C177	Odpowiedź słowna	Kōtō ni yoru aizu
C178	Znak dany ręką	Te ni yoru aizu
C179	Przycisk urządzenia sygnalizującego	Oshi-botan
C180	Brzęczyk	Shingō-on
C181	Zapis ręczny	Tegaki-kiroku
C182	Zapis półautomatyczny	Han-jidō-kiroku
C183	Zapis automatyczny	Jidō-kiroku
C184	Automatyzacja	Jidōka, Automation
C185	Program	Programme
C186	Perymetria komputerowa	Computer ni yoru shiyakeisoku
C187	Schemat wykresu	Kiroku zuhyō
C188	Skala wykresu	Zuhyō memori
C189	Połączenie wielokątne punktów izopteru	Chokusen-setsugō

	English	*Français*
C190	Fluent fitting (of isopter) by eye	Relier les points (d'un isoptère) par une courbe idéalisée
C191	Cartographic deformation	Déformation cartographique
C192	Polar azimuthal equidistant projection	Projection polaire azimuthale équidistante
C193	Central tangential projection	Projection centrale tangentielle
C194	Parabolic projection	Projection parabolique
C195	Equivalent projections	Projections équivalentes
C196	Conformal projections	Projections conformes
C197	To hatch	Hachurer
C198	Interpretation of a visual field chart	Interprétation d'un tracé périmétrique
C199	Area of a field defect	Surface d'un déficit
C200	Density of a field defect	Densité d'un déficit périmétrique
C201	Protocol	Protocole
C202	Control examination	Examen de contrôle
C203	Follow-up	Follow-up
C204	Data bank	Stockage de données
D0	**Normal visual field**	**Champ visuel normal**
D1	Ergoramic occupational visual field	Champ visuel ergoranomique
D2	Panoramic occupational visual field	Champ visuel panoramique
D3	Total dynamic field	Champ total dynamique
D4	Fixation point	Point de fixation
D5	Meridian	Méridien
D6	Parallel circle	Parallèle
D7	Central field	Champ central
D8	Midzone	Zone moyenne
D9	Periphery	Périphérie
D10	Hemifield	Hémichamp
D11	Quadrant	Quadrant

	Deutsch	Español
C190	idealisierte Verbindung der Isopterenmesspunkte	Unir los puntos (de una isóptera) por une curva idealizada
C191	kartographische Verzeichnung	Deformación cartográfica
C192	gleichabständig azimuthale Polarprojektion	Proyección polar azimutale equidistante
C193	zentrale Tangentenprojektion	Proyección central tangencial
C194	parabolische Projektion	Proyección parabólica
C195	gleichwertige Projektionen	Proyecciones equivalentes
C196	formgleiche Projektionen	Proyecciones conformes
C197	Schraffieren	Incubar
C198	Deutung eines Gesichtsfeldbefundes	Interpretación de un déficit perimétrico
C199	Ausfallsbereich	Superficie de un déficit perimétrico
C200	Skotomtiefe	Densidad de un déficit perimétrico
C201	Protokoll	Protocolo
C202	Kontrolluntersuchung	Examen de control
C203	Follow-up	Follow-up
C204	Datenspeicher	Deposito de datos
D0	**Normales Gesichtsfeld**	**Campo visual normal**
D1	Arbeitsgesichtsfeld	Campo visual ergorámico
D2	Orientierungsgesichtsfeld	Campo visual panorámico
D3	Umblickfeld	Campo total dinámico
D4	Fixationspunkt	Punto de fijación
D5	Meridian	Meridiano
D6	Parallelkreis	Paralelo
D7	zentrales Gesichtsfeld	Campo central
D8	Mittelzone	Zona media
D9	Peripherie	Periferia
D10	Gesichtsfeldhälfte	Hemicampo
D11	Quadrant	Cuadrante

	Russkii	*Italiano*
C190	Idealizirovannaia krivaia (izoptera)	Connessione curva ad occhio (dell'isottera)
C191	Kartograficheskaia deformatisiia	Deformazione cartografica
C192	Poliarnaia proektsiia s ravnootstoiashchimi azimutami	Proiezione polare equidistante azimutale
C193	Tsentral'naia tangentsial'naia proektsiia	Proiezione centrale tangenziale
C194	Parabolicheskaia proektsiia	Proiezione parabolica
C195	Ekvivalentnye proektsii	Proiezione equivalente
C196	Sootvetstvuiushchaia proektiia	Proiezione conforme
C197	Shtrikhovat'	Tratteggiare
C198	Interpretatsiia skhemy polia zreniia	Interpretazione di un tracciato di campo visivo
C199	Ploshchad' defecta polia zreniia	Superficie di un deficit perimetrico
C200	Plotnost' defecta polia zreniia	Densità di un deficit perimetrico
C201	Protokol	Protocollo
C202	Kontrol'noe issledovanie	Esame di controllo
C203	Proslezhivanie	Controllo successivo
C204	Arkhiv dannykh	Raccolta dei dati
D0	**Normal'noe pole zreniia**	**Campo visivo normale**
D1	Rabochee pole zreniia (professional'noe)	Campo visivo ergoramico (di lavoro)
D2	Pole zreniia panoramnoe (professional'noe)	Campo visivo panoramico
D3	Obshchee dinamicheskoe pole	Campo totale dinamico
D4	Tockha fiksatsii	Punto di fissazione
D5	Meridian	Meridiano
D6	Parellel'noe kol'tso	Cerchio parallelo
D7	Psentral'noe pole	Campo centrale
D8	Promezhutochnaia zona	Zona media
D9	Periferiia	Periferia
D10	Polovina polia	Emicampo
D11	Kvadrant	Quadrante

	Svenska	*Nederlands*
C190	Isopterkonstruktion på fri hand	Vloeiende afronding van de isopter
C191	Kartografisk deformation	Cartografische vervorming
C192	Polär azimutal ekvidistant projektion	Polaire azimutale gelijkmatige projectie
C193	Central tangentiell projektion	Centrale tangentiële projectie
C194	Parabolisk projektion	Parabolische projectie
C195	Ekvivalent projektion	Gelijkwaardige projecties
C196	Konformal projektion	Gelijkvormige projecties
C197	Streckning	Arceren
C198	Tolkning av synfältsdiagram	Interpretatie van een gezichtsveldtracé
C199	Yta av synfältsdefekt	Oppervlakte van een perimetrisch defect
C200	Djup av synfältsdefekt	Intensiteit van een perimetrisch defect
C201	Protokoll	Protocol
C202	Kontrollundersökning	Controle-onderzoek
C203	Uppföljning	Follow-up
C204	Databank	Opslagen van gegevens
D0	**Normalt synfält**	**Normaal gezichtsveld**
D1	Ergoramiskt synfält	Ergoramisch gezichtsveld
D2	Panoramiskt synfält	Panoramisch gezichtsveld
D3	Totalt dynamiskt fält	Veld van het rondkijken
D4	Fixationspunkt	Fixatiepunt
D5	Meridian	Meridiaan
D6	Parallellcirkel	Parallel
D7	Centralt fält	Centraal gezichtsveld
D8	Mittzon	Intermediair gezichtsveld
D9	Periferi	Periferie
D10	Hemifält	Gezichtsveldhelft
D11	Kvadrant	Kwadrant

	Polski	*Nihongo*
C190	Połączenie punktów izopteru w postaci gładkiej, krzywej linii	Kyokusen-setsugō
C191	Zniekształcenie kartograficzne	Seizu-jō no henkei
C192	Projekcja biegunowa, azymutowa o równych odstępach	Tōkyori-kyokuhōi tōsha
C193	Projekcja środkowa styczna	Chūshinbu-seisetsu tōsha
C194	Projekcja paraboliczna	Hōbutsusen tōsha
C195	Projekcja równowartościowa	Tōseki tōsha
C196	Projekcja o dostosowanej formie	Sōji tōsha
C197	kreskować	Shima-kage o tsukeru
C198	Interpretacja badania pola widzenia	Shiya-zukei no kaishaku
C199	Obszar ubytku perymetrycznego	Shiya-kesson-bu
C200	Głębokość ubytku perymetrycznego	Shiya-kesson no mitsudo
C201	Protokół	Protocol
C202	Badanie kontrolne	Taishō-jikken
C203	Obserwacja dalsza	Follow-up
C204	Bank danych	Dētā no chikuseki
D0	**Pole widzenia prawidłowe**	**Shiya**
D1	Pole widzenia ergoramiczne	Ergoramic visual field
D2	Pole widzenia panoramiczne	Panoramic visual field
D3	Pole widzenia dynamiczne	Umblickfeld
D4	Punkt fiksacji	Koshi-ten
D5	Południk	Keisen
D6	Koło równoległe	Heikosen, Isen
D7	Pole widzenia środkowe	Chūshin shiya
D8	Strefa środkowa	Chūkan-tai
D9	Obwód	Shūhen
D10	Pole widzenia połowicze	Nibun no ichi shiya (1/2)
D11	Kwadrant	Yonbun no ichi (1/4)

	English	*Français*
D12	temporal	temporal
D13	nasal	nasal
D14	superior	supérieur
D15	inferior	inférieur
D16	supero-temporal, etc.	temporal supérieur, etc.
D17	Eccentricity	Excentricité
D18	Absolute limits	Limites absolues
D19	Profile	Profil
D20	Isopter	Isoptère
D21	Central peak	Pic central
D22	Peripheral limits	Limites périphériques
D23	Blind spot	Tache aveugle
D24	Angioscotoma	Angioscotome
D25	Vertical asymmetry of the isopters	Asymétrie verticale des isoptères
D26	Central scotoma at low light levels	Scotome central à l'obscur
D27	Hemiopic border	Bord hémiopique
D28	Horizontal raphe	Raphé horizontal
D29	Refractive scotoma	Scotome de réfraction
D30	Rotation of the blind spot	Rotation de la tache aveugle
E0	**Pathology**	**Pathologie**
E1	Defect	Déficit
E2	Absolute defect	Déficit absolu
E3	Relative defect	Déficit relatif
E4	Chromatic defect	Déficit chromatique
E5	Gradient	Gradient
E6	Steep slope	Pente raide
E7	Gradual (= gentle) slope	Pente douce
E8	Notch	Encoche
E9	Peripheral defect	Déficit périphérique
E10	Contraction	Rétrécissement
E11	Concentric contraction	Rétrécissement concentrique
E12	Generalized concentric contraction	Rétrécissement concentrique généralisé
E13	Scotoma	Scotome
E14	Positive scotoma	Scotome positif
E15	Negative scotoma	Scotome négatif
E16	Depression of the sensitivity curve	Dépression de la courbe de sensibilité

	Deutsch	Español
D12	temporal	temporal
D13	nasal	nasal
D14	oberer	superior
D15	unterer	inferior
D16	temporal-oberer, usw.	temporal superior, etc.
D17	Exzentrizität	Excentricidad
D18	absolute Grenzen	Límites absolutos
D19	Profil	Perfil
D20	Isoptere	Isóptera
D21	zentrale Spitze	Pico central
D22	periphere Grenzen	Limites periféricos
D23	blinder Fleck	Mancha ciega
D24	Angioskotom	Angio-escotoma
D25	vertikale Asymmetrie der Isopteren	Asimetría vertical de las isópteras
D26	zentrales Dunkelskotom	Escotoma central al oscuro
D27	Halbseitengrenze	Borde hemiópico
D28	Horizontale Raphe	Rafe horizontal
D29	Refraktionskotom	Escotoma de refracción
D30	Verrollung des blinden Fleckes	Translado circular de la mancha ciega
E0	**Pathologie**	**Patología**
E1	Ausfall	Déficit
E2	absoluter Ausfall	Déficit absoluto
E3	relativer Ausfall	Déficit relativo
E4	Ausfall für Farbwahrnehmung	Déficit cromático
E5	Gefälle	Gradiente
E6	steiles Gefälle	Pendiente abrupta
E7	flaches Gefälle	Pendiente suave
E8	Kerbe, Eindellung	Entrada
E9	peripherer Ausfall	Déficit periférico
E10	Einengung	Estrechamiento
E11	konzentrische Einengung	Estrechamiento concéntrico
E12	allgemeine konzentrische Einengung	Estrechamiento concentrico generalizado
E13	Skotom	Escotoma
E14	positives Skotom	Escotoma positivo
E15	negatives Skotom	Escotoma negativo
E16	Herabsetzung der Empfindlichkeitskurve	Depresión

	Russkii	*Italiano*
D12	visochnyi	temporale
D13	nosovoi	nasale
D14	verkhnii	superiore
D15	nizhinii	inferiore
D16	verkhne-visochnyi	temporale superiore, etc.
D17	Ekstsentrisitet	Eccentricità
D18	Absoliutnye granitsy	Limite assoluto
D19	Profil'	Profilo
D20	Izoptera	Isottera
D21	Tsentral'nyi pik	Picco centrale
D22	Perifericheskie granitsy	Limite periferico
D23	Slepoe piatno	Macchia cieca
D24	Angioskotoma	Angioscotoma
D25	Vertikal'naia asimmetria izopter	Asimmetrica verticale delle isoptere
D26	Tsentral'naia skotoma pri slabom svete	Scotoma centrale a bassa intensità luminosa
D27	Gemiopicheskii krai (granitsa)	Bordo emianoptico
D28	Gorizontal'nyi shov	Rafe orizzontale
D29	Refraktsionnaia skotoma	Scotoma di refrazione
D30	Vrashchenie slepogo piatna	Traslazione circolare della macchia cieca
E0	**Patologiia**	**Patologia**
E1	Defekt	Deficit
E2	Absoliutnyi defekt	Deficit assoluto
E3	Otnositel'nyi defekt	Deficit relativo
E4	Khromaticheskii defekt	Deficit cromatico
E5	Gradient	Gradiente
E6	Krutoi skat	Pendenza ripida
E7	Pologii skat	Pendenza dolce
E8	Vyemka (vyrezka)	Tacca
E9	Perifericheskii defekt	Deficit periferico
E10	Suzhenie	Restringimento
E11	Kontsentricheskoe suzhenie	Restringimento concentrico
E12	Generalizovannoe kontsentricheskoe suzhenie	Restringimento concentrico generalizzato
E13	Skotoma	Scotoma
E14	Polozhitel'naia skotoma	Scotoma positivo
E15	Otritsatel'naia skotoma	Scotoma negativo
E16	Snizhenie (podavlenie) krivoi chuvstvitel'nosti	Depressione della curva di sensibilità

	Svenska	*Nederlands*
D12	temporal	temporaal
D13	nasal	nasaal
D14	övre	bovenste
D15	undre	onderste
D16	övre temporal, etc.	bovenste temporaal, enz.
D17	Excentricitet	Excentriciteit
D18	Absoluta gränser	Absolute grenzen
D19	Profil	Profiel
D20	Isopter	Isopter
D21	Central topp	Centrale top
D22	Perifera gränser	Perifere grenzen
D23	Blind fläck	Blinde vlek
D24	Kärlskotom	Angioscotoom
D25	Vertikal isopterasymmetri	Vertikale asymmetrie van de isopteren
D26	Centralskotom i dunkel belysning	Centraal scotoom in de duisternis
D27	Hemiopisk gräns	Hemiopische rand
D28	Horisontellt band	Horizontale raphe
D29	Refraktionsskotom	Refractiescotoom
D30	Rotation av blinda fläcken	Rotatie van de blinde vlek
E0	**Patologi**	**Pathologie**
E1	Defekt	Defect
E2	Absolut defekt	Absoluut defect
E3	Relativ defekt	Relatief defect
E4	Kromatisk defekt	Chromatisch defect
E5	Sluttning	Gradiënt
E6	Brant sluttning	Steile helling
E7	Liten sluttning	Zachte helling
E8	Hack	Inkeping
E9	Perifer defekt	Perifeer defect
E10	Kontraktion	Vernauwing
E11	Koncentrisk kontraktion	Concentrische vernauwing
E12	Generell koncentrisk kontraktion	Veralgemeende concentrische vernauwing
E13	Skotom	Scotoom
E14	Positivt skotom	Positief scotoom
E15	Negativt skotom	Negatief scotoom
E16	Sänkning av känslighetskurvan	Verlaging van de gevoeligheidscurve

	Polski	*Nihongo*
D12	skroniowy	Jisoku
D13	nosowy	Bisoku
D14	górny	Jō
D15	dolny	Ka
D16	skroniowo-górny	Jō-jisoku
D17	Odśrodkowość	Henshindo
D18	Granice absolutne	Zettai genkai
D19	Profil	Danmen
D20	Izopter	Tōkandosen
D21	Szczytśrodkowy	Chushin no peak
D22	Granice obwodowe	Shūhen no genkai
D23	Plama ślepa	Mōten
D24	Mroczek naczyniowy	Kekkan-anten
D25	Asymetria pionowa izopterów	Tōkandosen no suichoku hitaishō
D26	Mroczek środkowy dla niskich wartości światła	Teishōdo no chushin anten
D27	Granica niedowidzenia połowiczego	Hanmō no kyōkai
D28	Szew poziomy	Suihei hō sen
D29	Mroczek refrakcyjny	Kussetsusei anten
D30	Rotacja plamy ślepej	Mōten no kaisen
E0	**Patologia**	**Byōri**
E1	Ubytek	Kesson
E2	Ubytek bezwzględny	Zettai
E3	Ubytek wzlędny	Hikaku
E4	Ubytek dla barw	Shikisai
E5	Gradient	Kōbai
E6	Spadek stromy	Kyū na kōbai
E7	Spadek stopniowy	Yuruyaka na kōbai
E8	Wrąb	Sekkon, saikon
E9	Ubytek obwodowy	Shūhen kesson
E10	Zawężenie	Kyōsaku
E11	Zawężenie współśrodkowe	Dōshinsei kyōsaku
E12	Zawężenie współśrodkowe uogólnione	Zenpanteki na dōshinsei kyōsaku
E13	Mroczek	Anten
E14	Mroczek pozytywny	Jissei anten
E15	Mroczek negatywny	Kyosei anten
E16	Obniżenie krzywej wrażliwości	Kandokyokusen no teika

	English	*Français*
E17	Central scotoma	Scotome central
E18	Eccentric fixation	Fixation excentrique
E19	Eccentric viewing	Vision excentrique
E20	Displacement of the blind spot	Déplacement de la tache aveugle
E21	Macular scotoma	Scotome maculaire
E22	Scotoma caused by inhibition	Scotome d'inhibition
E23	Paracentral scotoma	Scotome paracentral
E24	Pericentral scotoma	Scotome péricentral
E25	Paracaecal scotoma	Scotome paracaecal
E26	Pericaecal scotoma (= enlargement of the blind spot)	Scotome péricaecal (= agrandissement de la tache aveugle)
E27	Baring of the blind spot	Exclusion de la tache aveugle
E28	Centrocaecal scotoma	Scotome caecocentral
E29	Ring scotoma	Scotome annulaire
E30	Zonular scotoma	Scotome zonulaire (= en ceinture)
E31	Nerve fibre(er)s bundle defect (= NFBD)	Déficit fasciculaire (= DF)
E32	Central NFBD	DF central
E33	Juxta-papillary NFBD	DF juxtacaecal
E34	Arcuate NFBD (= Bjerrum scotoma)	DF arciforme (= scotome de Bjerrum)
E35	A NFBD in a nasal quadrant	DF d'un quadrant nasal
E36	A NFBD in a temporal quadrant	DF d'un quadrant temporal
E37	Cuneate NFBD	DF cunéiforme
E38	NFBD proceeding away from the blind spot	DF caecofugal
E39	NFBD proceeding towards the blind spot	DF caecopétal
E40	Break through	Break through
E41	Swiss cheese defect, Sieve-like defect	Déficit en fromage de Gruyère

	Deutsch	*Español*
E17	Zentralskotom	Escotoma central
E18	exzentrische Fixation	Fijación excéntrica
E19	exzentrisches Sehen	Visión excéntrica
E20	Verlagerung des blinden Fleckes	Desplazamiento de la mancha ciega
E21	maculares Skotom	Escotoma macular
E22	Hemmungsskotom	Escotoma de inhibición
E23	parazentrales Skotom	Escotoma para-central
E24	perizentrales Skotom	Escotoma peri-central
E25	paracoecales Skotom	Escotoma para-cecal
E26	pericoecales Skotom (= Vergrösserung des blinden Fleckes)	Escotoma peri-cecal (= agrandamiento de la mancha ciega)
E27	Ausparung des blinden Fleckes	Exclusión de la mancha ciega
E28	zentrocoecales Skotom	Escotoma ceco-central
E29	parazentrales Ringskotom	Escotoma anular
E30	peripheres Ringskotom	Escotoma zonular (= en cinturón)
E31	NervenfaserbündelAusfall (= NFBA)	Déficit fascicular (= DF)
E32	zentraler NFBA	DF central
E33	juxtapapillärer NFBA	DF yuxtacecal
E34	Bogenskotom (= Bjerrum-Skotom)	DF arciforme (= escotoma de Bjerrum)
E35	NFBA in einem nasalen Quadranten	DF de un cuadrante nasal
E36	NFBA in einem temporalen Quadranten	DF de un cuadrante temporal
E37	keilförmiger NFBA	DF cuneiforme
E38	coecofugaler NFBA	DF ceco-fugal
E39	coecopetaler NFBA	DF ceco-petal
E40	Durchbruch	Break through
E41	Siebförmiger Defekt	Déficit en queso gruyere

	Russkii	*Italiano*
E17	Tsentral'naia skotoma	Scotoma centrale
E18	Ekstsentricheskaia fiksatsiia	Fissazione eccentrica
E19	Ekstsentricheskoe zrenie	Visione eccentrica
E20	Smeshchenie slepogo piatna	Spostamento della macchia cieca
E21	Makuliarnaia skotoma	Scotoma maculare
E22	Skotoma, obuslovlennaia tormozheniem	Scotoma d'inibizione
E23	Paratsentral'naia skotoma	Scotoma paracentrale
E24	Peritsentral'naia skotoma	Scotoma pericentrale
E25	Paratsekal'naia skotoma	Scotoma paracecale
E26	Peritsekal'naia skotoma (= uvelichenie slepogo piatna)	Scotoma pericecale (= ingrandimento della macchia cieca)
E27	Vykliuchenie (obnazhenie) slepogo piatna	Esclusione della macchia cieca
E28	Tsentrotsekal'naia skotoma	Scotoma ciecocentrale
E29	Kol'tsevaia skotoma	Scotoma anulare
E30	Zonuliarnaia skotoma	Scotoma zonulare (= a cintura)
E31	Defekt vsledstvie porazheniia puchkov nervnykh volokon (DPPNV)	Deficit fascicolato (= DF)
E32	Tsentral'nyi DPPNV	DF centrale
E33	Iuksta-papilliarnyi DPPNV	DF justaciecale
E34	Dugovoi DPPNV (= Skotoma B'erruma)	DF arciforme (= scotoma di Bjerrum)
E35	DPPNV nazalonogo kvadranta	DF d'un quadrante nasale
E36	DPPNV visochnogo kvadranta	DF di un quadrante temporale
E37	Klinovidnyi DPPNV	DF cuneiforme
E38	Tsekofugal'nyi DPPNV	DF ciecofugale
E39	Tsekopetal'nyi DPPNV	DF ciecopetale
E40	Proryv skotomy	Rottura attraverso
E41	Skotoma po tipu "shveitsarskii syr"	Difetto a formaggio svizzero

	Svenska	Nederlands
E17	Centralskotom	Centraal scotoom
E18	Excentrisk fixation	Excentrische fixatie
E19	Excentrisk blick	Excentrisch zien
E20	Förskjutning av blinda fläcken	Verplaatsing van de blinde vlek
E21	Makulärt skotom	Maculair scotoom
E22	Inhibitionsskotom	Inhibitiescotoom
E23	Paracentralt skotom	Paracentraal scotoom
E24	Pericentralt skotom	Pericentraal scotoom
E25	Paracekalt skotom	Paracaecaal scotoom
E26	Pericekalt skotom (= förstorad blind fläck)	Pericaecaal scotoom (= vergroting van de blinde vlek)
E27	Baring of the blind spot	Uitsluiting van de blinde vlek
E28	Centrocekalt skotom	Caeco-centraal scotoom
E29	Ringskotom	Ringscotoom
E30	Zonulärt skotom	Gordelscotoom
E31	Nervfiberbuntdefekt (= NFBD)	Bundeldefect (= BD)
E32	Central NFBD	Centraal BD
E33	Juxtapapillär NFBD	Juxtacaecaal BD
E34	Arcuat NFBD (= Bjerrumskotom)	Arciform BD (= Bjerrumscotoom)
E35	Nasal NFBD	BD van een nasaal kwadrant
E36	Temporal NFBD	BD van een temporaal kwadrant
E37	Kilformad NFBD	Wigvormig BD
E38	NFBD riktad från blinda fläcken	Caecofugaal BD
E39	NFBD riktad mot blinda fläcken	Caecopetaal BD
E40	Genombrott	Doorbraak
E41	Schweizerostdefekt	Zeefscotoom

	Polski	*Nihongo*
E17	Mroczek środkowy	Chūshin anten
E18	Fiksacja ekscentryczna	Chūshin gai koshi
E19	Widzenie ekscentryczna	Chūshin gai shi
E20	Przemieszczenie plamy ślepej	Mōten no ten-i
E21	Mroczek plamkowy	Ōhan-anten
E22	Mroczek uwarunkowany tłumieniem	Yokusei anten
E23	Mroczek przyśrodkowy	Chūshin gai anten
E24	Mroczek okołośrodkowy	Bō chushin anten
E25	Mroczek przy plamie ślepej	Bō mōten anten
E26	Mroczek wokół plamy ślepej (= powiększenie plamy ślepej)	Mōten no kakudai
E27	Ogołocenie plamy ślepej	Mōten no roshutsu
E28	Mroczek środkowy łączący się z plamą ślepą	Mōten chūshin anten
E29	Mroczek obrączkowy	Rinjō anten
E30	Mroczek pierścieniowy obwodowy	Taijō anten
E31	Uszkodzenie pęczka włókien nerwowych (= UPWN)	Sokujō anten (SA)
E32	UPWN środkowe	Chūshin SA
E33	UPWN przytarczowe	Bo mohan SA
E34	UPWN łukowate (= mroczek Bjerum'a)	Kyū-jō anten
E35	UPWN w kwadrancie skroniowym	Bisoku 1/4 SA
E36		Jisoku 1/4 SA
E37	UPWN wycinkowe	Kitsujō SA
E38	UPWN odchodzące od plamy ślepej	Mohan yori hirogaru SA
E39	UPWN powiększające się w kierunku plamy ślepej	Mohan e mukau SA
E40	Połączenie się mroczka z obwodem pola	Shadan suru
E41	Ubytek podobny do sera szwajcarskiego	Swiss cheese defect

	English	*Français*
E42	Defect of vascular origin	Déficit d'origine vasculaire
E43	Neuroscotoma	Neuroscotome
E44	Hemianopia	Hémianopsie
E45	hemianopic	hémianopique
E46	Hemidysopia (= relative hemianopia)	Hémidysopsie (= hémianopsie relative)
E47	Hemiachromatopsia	Hémiachromatopsie
E48	Quadrantanopia	Quadranopsie
		en quadrant
E49	quadrantic	
E50	Quadrant dysopia (= relative quadrantanopia)	Dysopsie en quadrant (= quadranopsie relative)
E51	heteronymous	hétéronyme
E52	bitemporal	bitemporale
E53	binasal	binasale
E54	homonymous	homonyme
E55	left	gauche
E56	right	droite
E57	vertical	verticale
E58	horizontal	horizontale
E59	crossed	croisée
E60	Step (nasal etc.)	Ressaut (nasal etc.)
E61	Hemianopic central scotoma (heteronymous-, etc.)	Scotome central hémianopique (hétéronyme, etc.)
E62	Quadrantanopic central scotoma (id.)	Scotome central quadranopique (id.)
E63	Symmetrical defect	Déficit symétrique
E64	Asymmetrical defect	Déficit asymétrique
E65	Congruent defect	Déficit congruent
E66	Incongruent defect	Déficit incongruent
E67	Temporal crescent	Faucille temporale
E68	Overshot	Overshot

	Deutsch	Español
E42	vasculär-bedingter Ausfall	Déficit de origen vascular
E43	Neuroskotom	Neuro-escotoma
E44	Hemianopsie	Hemianópsia
E45	hemianopisch	hemianópico
E46	Hemidysopsie (= relative Hemianopsie)	Hemidisópsia (= hemianópsia relativa)
E47	Halbseiten-Farbenblindkeit	Hemi-acromatópsia
E48	Quadrantenanopsie	Quadrantópsia en cuadrante
E49	quadrantenförmig	
E50	Quadrantendysopsie (= relative Quadrantenanopsie)	Disópsia en cuadrante (= quadrantópsia relativa)
E51	heteronym	heterónimo
E52	bitemporal	bitemporal
E53	binasal	binasal
E54	homonym	homónimo
E55	link(-er usw.)	izquierdo
E56	recht(-er usw.)	derecho
E57	vertikal	vertical
E58	horizontal	horizontal
E59	gekreuzt	cruzada
E60	Sprung (nasaler usw.)	Escalón (nasal, etc.)
E61	hemianopisches Zentralskotom (heteronymes, usw.)	Escotoma central hemianópsico (heteronimo, etc.)
E62	quadrantenanopisches Zentralskotom (ebenso)	Escotoma central en cuadrante (etc.)
E63	symmetrischer Ausfall	Déficit simétrico
E64	asymmetrischer Ausfall	Déficit asimétrico
E65	kongruenter Ausfall	Déficit congruente
E66	inkongruenter Ausfall	Déficit incongruente
E67	Gianuzzi'scher Halbmond	Semiluna temporal
E68	Überschuss	Overshot

	Russkii	*Italiano*
E42	Defekt sosudistoi prirody (proiskhozhdeniia)	Deficit vascolare
E43	Neiroskotoma	Neuroscotoma
E44	Gemianopiia	Emianopsia
E45	gemianopicheskii	emianopico
E46	Gemidizopiia (= otnositel'-naia gemianopiia)	Emidisopsia (= emianopsia relativa)
E47	Gemiakhromatopsiia	Emiacromatopsia
E48	Kvadrantanopiia	Quadranopsia quadrante
E49	kvadrantnyi	
E50	Kvadrantnaia dizopiia (= otnositel'naia kvadrantanopiia)	Disopsia a quadrante (= quadranopsia relativa)
E51	geteronimnyi	eteronimo
E52	bitemporal'nyi	bitemporale
E53	binazal'nyi	binasale
E54	gomonimnyi	omonimo
E55	levyi	sinistro
E56	pravyi	destro
E57	vertikal'nyi	verticale
E58	gorizontal'nyi	orizzontale
E59	perekreshchennyi	crociato
E60	"Stupen'ka" (nosovaia i dr.)	Gradino (nasale, ecc.)
E61	Gemianopicheskaia tsentral'naia skotoma (geteronimnaia i t.d.)	Scotoma centrale emianopico (eteronimo, ecc.)
E62	Kvadrantanopicheskaia tsentral'naia skotoma (i t.d.)	Scotoma centrale quadranopico (id.)
E63	Simmetrichnyi defekt	Deficit simmetrico
E64	Asimmetrichnyi defekt	Deficit asimmetrico
E65	Kongruentnyi (sovpadaiushchii) defekt	Deficit congruente
E66	Nesovpadaiushchii defekt	Deficit incongrente
E67	Visochnyi polumesiats	Falce temporale
E68	Promakhivanie	Overshot

	Svenska	Nederlands
E42	Defekt med vaskulär genes	Vasculair defect
E43	Neuroskotom	Neuroscotoom
E44	Hemianopsi	Hemianopsie
E45	hemianopsisk	hemianopisch
E46	Hemidysopsi (= relativ hemidefekt)	Hemidysopsie (= relatieve hemianopie)
E47	Hemidyskromatopsi	Hemiachromatopsie
E48	Kvadrantanopsi	Kwadranopsie
E49	kvadrantisk	in kwadrant
E50	Kvadrantdysopsi (= relativ kvadrantdefekt)	Kwadrant-dysopsie (= relatieve kwadranopsie)
E51	heteronym	heteroniem
E52	bitemporal	bitemporaal
E53	binasal	binasaal
E54	homonym	homoniem
E55	vänster	linker
E56	höger	rechter
E57	vertikal	vertikaal
E58	horisontell	horizontaal
E59	korsad	gekruist
E60	Steg (nasalt, etc)	(Nasale enz.) Sprong
E61	Hemianopiskt centralskotom (heteronymt, etc.)	Hemianopisch centraal scotoom (heteroniem-, enz.)
E62	Kvadrantanopiskt centralskotom (etc.)	Kwadranopisch centraal scotoom (enz.)
E63	Symmetrisk defekt	Symmetrisch defect
E64	Asymmetrisk defekt	Asymmetrisch defect
E65	Kongruent defekt	Congruënt defect
E66	Inkongruent defekt	Incongruënt defect
E67	Temporal skära	Monoculaire temporale sikkel
E68	Overshot	Overshot

	Polski	*Nihongo*
E42	Ubytek uwarunkowany zmianami naczyniowymi	Kekkan sei anten
E43	Mroczek środkowy uwarunkowany UPWN	Neuroscotoma
E44	Niedowidzenie połowicze	Han-mō
E45	połowiczo-niedowidzący	Han-mō-sei
E46	Hemianopsja (= niedowidzenie połowicze względne)	Hikaku hanmō
E47	Niedowidzenie połowicze dla barw	Hemiachromatopsia
E48	Niedowidzenie kwadrantowe	Yonbun no ichi hanmō
E49	kwadrantowy	Yonbun no ichi no
E50	Dysopsja kwadrantowa	1/4 hikaku han-mō
E51	różnoimienny	Imei no
E52	dwuskroniowy	Ryō-jisoku
E53	dwunosowy	Ryō-bisoku
E54	jednoimienny	Dōmei no
E55	lewy	Hidari
E56	prawy	Migi
E57	pionowy	Suichoku no
E58	poziomy	Suihei no
E59	skrzyżowany	Kōsasei no
E60	Schód (nosowy itd.)	Dankai, Step
E61	Mroczek środkowy połowiczy (różnoimienny itd.)	Hanmō sei chūshin anten (Imeisei nado)
E62	Mroczek środkowy kwadrantowy	1/4 hanmō sei chūshin anten
E63	Ubytek symetryczny	Taishō sei kesson
E64	Ubytek asymetryczny	Hi-taisho sei kesson
E65	Ubytek zgodny	Icchi suru kesson
E66	Ubytek niezgodny	Fu-icchi kesson
E67	Półksiężyc skroniowy	Jisoku-hangetsujō tangan shiya
E68	"Nadmiar" (resztkowe pole widzenia większe niż typowo)	Overshot

	English	*Français*
E69	Sparing of the macula	Epargne maculaire
E70	Splitting of the macula	Division maculaire
E71	Agnosia	Agnosie
E72	Cortical blindness	Cécité corticale
E73	Handicap	Handicap
E74	Degree of disability	Degré d'invalidité
E75	one-eyed	borgne
E76	Esterman grid	Grille d'Esterman
E77	Enlargement of a field defect	Augmentation d'un déficit périmétrique
E78	Diminution of a field defect	Diminution d'un déficit périmétrique
E79	Disappearance of a field defect	Disparition d'un déficit périmétrique
E80	Malingering (or simulation) of a field defect	Simulation d'un déficit périmétrique
E81	Hysterical field defect	Déficit périmétrique hystérique
E82	Concealment of a field defect	Dissimulation d'un déficit périmétrique

	Deutsch	Español
E69	Maculaausparung	Respeto macular
E70	Maculahalbierung	División macular
E71	Agnosie	Agnosia
E72	Rindenblindheit	Ceguera cortical
E73	Behinderung	Handicap
E74	Erwerbsminderung einäugige	Grado de invalidez mono-vidente
E75	Esterman-Gitter	Grilla de Esterman
E76	Vergrösserung eines Gesichtsfeldausfalles	Aumento de un déficit perimétrico
E77	Verkleinerung eines Gesichtsfeldausfalles	Disminución de un déficit perimétrico
E78	Verschwinden einen Gesichtsfeldausfalles	Desaparición de un déficit perimétrico
E79	Simulation eines Gesichtsfeldausfalles	Simulación de un déficit périmétrico
E80	hysterischer Gesichtsfeldausfall	Déficit perimétrico histérico
E81	Dissimulation eines Gesichtsfeldausfalles	Disimulación de un déficit perimétrico

	Russkii	*Italiano*
E69	Sokhrannost' makuly	Risparmio maculare
E70	Rasshcheplenie makuly	Divisione maculare
E71	Agnoziia	Agnosia
E72	Kortikal'naia slepota	Cecità corticale
E73	Gandikap	Handicap
E74	Stepen' invalidizatsii	Grado di invalidità
E75	Odnoglazyi	cieco da un occhio
E76	Reshetka Estermana	Griglia di Esterman
E77	Uvelichenie ploshchadi defekta	Allargamento di un deficit perimetrico
E78	Umen'skenie ploshchadi defekta	Diminuzione di un deficit perimetrico
E79	Ischeznovenie defekta polia zreniia	Scomparsa di un deficit perimetrico
E80	Simuliatsiia defekta polia zreniia	Simulazione di un deficit perimetrico
E81	Istericheskii defekt polia zreniia	Deficit perimetrico isterico
E82	Dissimuliatsiia perimetricheskogo defekta	Occultamento di un deficit perimetrico.

	Svenska	Nederlands
E69	Makula-sparning	Maculaire uitsparing
E70	Makula-delning	Splijting van de macula
E71	Agnosi	Agnosie
E72	Kortikal blindhet	Corticale blindheid
E73	Handikapp	Handicap
E74	Grad av handikapp	Invaliditeitsgraad
E75	Enögd	Eenogig
E76	Esterman-nät	Schema van Esterman
E77	Förstoring av synfälts-defekt	Toename van een perimetrisch defect
E78	Förminskning av synfälts-defekt	Afname van een perimetrisch defect
E79	Normalisering av synfälts-defekt	Verdwijning van een perimetrisch defect
E80	Simulering av synfältsde-fekt	Simulatie van een perimetrisch defect
E81	Hysterisk synfältsdefekt	Hysterisch perimetrisch defect
E82	Dissimulering av synfälts-defekt	Dissimulatie van een perimetrisch defect

	Polski	*Nihongo*
E69	Oszczędzenie plamki	Ōhan-kaihi
E70	Ubytek połowiczy plamkowy	Ōhan-bunkatsu
E71	Agnozja	Shitsu-nin
E72	Ślepota korowa	Hishitsu-mō
E73	Trudność (utrudnienie)	Handicap
E74	Stopień obniżenia sprawności do pracy	Haishitsu-do
E75	Jednooczny	Hengan no
E76	Siatka Esterman'a	Esterman no kōshi
E77	Powiększenie się ubytku perymetrycznego	Shiyakesson no kakudai
E78	Zmniejszenie się ubytku perymetrycznego	Shiyakesson no genshō
E79	Znikanie ubytku perymetrycznego	Shiyakesson no shōshitsu
E80	Symulowanie ubytku perymetrycznego	Sabyō sei shiyakesson
E81	Ubytek histeryczny w polu widzenia	Histery sei shiyakesson
E82	Dysymulowanie ubytku perymetrycznego	Shiyakesson no yūgō

Alphabetical list of the English terms

GPSR Compliance

The European Union's (EU) General Product Safety Regulation (GPSR) is a set of rules that requires consumer products to be safe and our obligations to ensure this.

If you have any concerns about our products, you can contact us on ProductSafety@springernature.com

In case Publisher is established outside the EU, the EU authorized representative is:

Springer Nature Customer Service Center GmbH
Europaplatz 3
69115 Heidelberg, Germany

Batch number: 10830943

Printed by Printforce, the Netherlands